AF432036

Cognitive Neuroscience & Neuropsychology

-

The Comprehensive Guide

by

VIRUTI SHIVAN

Masters in Clinical Psychology (Major)

"In books, as in life, it's not the size or looks but the content that matters."

Introduction

Welcome to "Cognitive Neuroscience & Neuropsychology - The Comprehensive Guide," a journey into the fascinating world of the brain and mind. This book is designed to bridge the gap between the complexity of neuroscientific research and the curiosity of those eager to understand the underpinnings of cognitive behavior and neuropsychological functioning. As we embark on this exploration, we delve into how our brains perceive, understand, and interact with the world around us.

Cognitive neuroscience and neuropsychology stand at the crossroads of several disciplines, combining insights from psychology, biology, medicine, and even philosophy to answer profound questions about human thought, emotion, and behavior. This book aims to provide a comprehensive overview of these fields, offering readers a solid foundation for understanding the mechanisms governing the mind and its processes.

The Absence of Visual Aids

Notably, this book does not contain images or illustrations. This decision was made not only for copyright reasons but also to challenge and engage the reader's imagination and conceptual understanding. We aim to paint a vivid picture of cognitive processes and brain functions through descriptive narratives and conceptual explanations, allowing the mind's eye to visualize what cannot be directly seen.

A Guide Through Complexity

Each chapter of this book is structured to unfold the complex layers of cognitive neuroscience and neuropsychology gradually. Starting with the basic building blocks of neural communication, we journey through the intricacies of sensation and perception, delve into the mysteries of memory and consciousness, and explore the profound impact of neurodevelopmental and neuropsychological disorders. The chapters are designed to be both standalone resources and parts of a cohesive whole, providing flexibility in how the material can be approached and understood.

Engagement Through Questions

At the end of each chapter, you will find exercises like multiple-choice questions (MCQs) with answers provided at the book's conclusion. These exercises are crafted to test comprehension, encourage critical thinking, and solidify the knowledge gained through each chapter. They serve as a tool for self-assessment and deeper engagement with the material.

Conclusion

As we proceed, remember that this book is more than just a collection of facts and theories. It is an invitation to think deeply about the human mind's and brain's marvels. It encourages readers to question, explore, and imagine cognitive neuroscience and neuropsychology's possibilities for understanding our essence. Whether you are a student, a professional in the field, or simply a curious mind, this guide is your portal to a deeper appreciation of the cognitive and neural dynamics that make us who we are. Let us embark on this enlightening journey with open minds and a keen curiosity.

Chapter 1: Foundations of Cognitive Neuroscience

1.1 The Evolution of Cognitive Neuroscience

Cognitive neuroscience, a term that harmonizes the expansive fields of cognition, brain, and behavior, traces its origins to a rich history of interdisciplinary research and curiosity about the human mind. This chapter delves into the evolutionary path of cognitive neuroscience, highlighting pivotal discoveries and theoretical shifts that have shaped our understanding of the brain's role in cognitive functions.

The Convergence of Disciplines

The birth of cognitive neuroscience can be attributed to the convergence of several scientific disciplines, each bringing its unique perspective on how the brain processes information. In the mid-20th century, researchers from psychology, neurobiology, computer science, and medicine began to merge their insights, driven by a common goal: to understand the neural underpinnings of thought, memory, perception, and emotion. This interdisciplinary approach was revolutionary, marking a departure from traditional studies that either focused on behavior (psychology) or the brain's physical structure (neurobiology) without considering how these elements interact.

Technological Advancements and Methodological Innovations

The advent of advanced neuroimaging technologies significantly accelerates the evolution of cognitive neuroscience. Techniques such as functional Magnetic Resonance Imaging (fMRI) and Positron Emission Tomography (PET) provided scientists with the tools to observe the brain in action, linking specific cognitive functions to distinct brain regions. This ability to visualize brain activity during cognitive tasks offered unprecedented insights into the dynamic nature of neural processing, fundamentally altering our understanding of brain function and organization.

Theoretical Milestones

Cognitive neuroscience has been shaped by several vital theoretical milestones throughout its evolution. For instance, the concept of neural plasticity challenged the once-static view of the brain, suggesting that neural connections could change in response to experience and learning. Another landmark theory, the modular organization of the brain, proposed that specific cognitive functions could be attributed to particular brain areas, leading to the identification of language centers, memory storage sites, and more. These theories, among others, have provided a framework for understanding the complexity of brain function and its relationship with cognitive processes.

The Role of Cognitive Psychology

Cognitive psychology, with its focus on the mechanisms of thought and knowledge, has played a crucial role in the development of cognitive neuroscience. Cognitive psychologists have offered testable hypotheses about the neural basis of mental processes by providing detailed models of cognition. This synergy between cognitive psychology and neuroscience has led to a deeper understanding of how abstract cognitive functions, such as decision-making and problem-solving, are grounded in physical neural networks.

Looking Forward

As we stand on the shoulders of giants, the evolution of cognitive neuroscience continues to be driven by technological innovations, theoretical advances, and interdisciplinary collaboration. The field is a testament to humanity's quest to understand the essence of thought, emotion, and consciousness. By tracing its historical roots, we gain a deeper appreciation for the complexity of the human brain and insight into the future directions of cognitive neuroscience research. The journey through the evolution of cognitive neuroscience is a reminder of the power of curiosity and the endless possibilities that arise from seeking to understand the mind's mysteries.

1.2 Key Concepts and Terms

As we delve deeper into cognitive neuroscience, it becomes essential to familiarize ourselves with the key concepts and terms that form the foundation of this interdisciplinary field. Understanding these terms enhances comprehension of the material presented in this guide and facilitates an appreciation for the nuances of cognitive and neural mechanisms. This section introduces and explains fundamental concepts and terms critical to studying cognitive neuroscience.

Neurons and Synapses

At the heart of cognitive neuroscience are neurons, the basic building blocks of the nervous system. Neurons are specialized cells responsible for transmitting information throughout the brain and body. Communication between neurons occurs via synapses, junctions where one neuron's axon terminal connects to another's dendrite. This synaptic transmission is the basis for all neural activity, including thought, emotion, and movement.

Neurotransmitters

Neurotransmitters are chemical messengers released by neurons to communicate across synapses. They can have excitatory or inhibitory effects on the receiving neuron, influencing whether it will generate a neural impulse. Key neurotransmitters include dopamine, serotonin, and acetylcholine, each playing crucial roles in regulating mood, arousal, attention, and memory.

Plasticity

Neural plasticity, or neuroplasticity, refers to the brain's ability to change and adapt due to experience. This includes the formation of new neural connections and the strengthening or weakening of existing ones. Plasticity is fundamental to learning, memory, and recovery from brain injury.

Cognitive Functions

Cognitive functions are mental processes that allow us to carry out any task from the simplest to the most complex. These include perception, attention, memory, language, problem-solving, and decision-making. Cognitive neuroscience aims to understand how these functions are implemented in the brain.

Brain Imaging Techniques

Brain imaging techniques are non-invasive methods to visualize and measure brain activity and structure. Prominent examples include:

- **Functional Magnetic Resonance Imaging (fMRI):** Measures brain activity by detecting changes in blood flow, offering insights into the brain regions involved in specific cognitive tasks.

- **Electroencephalography (EEG):** Records electrical activity in the brain, providing detailed information about the timing of brain responses to stimuli.

- **Positron Emission Tomography (PET):** Uses radioactive tracers to visualize how your brain uses glucose, indicating high activity areas during tasks.

Cortical and Subcortical Structures

The brain is divided into cortical and subcortical structures. The cerebral cortex, or simply cortex, is the outer layer of the brain, involved in high-level cognitive functions such as thought, language, and consciousness. Subcortical structures beneath the cortex affect emotion, memory, and automatic functions. Critical structures include the hippocampus, amygdala, thalamus, and basal ganglia.

Hemispheric Lateralization

Hemispheric lateralization refers to the tendency for some cognitive functions to be more dominant in one brain hemisphere than the other. For example, in most right-handed individuals, language processing is predominantly located in the left hemisphere, while spatial reasoning tends to be more right-hemisphere dominant.

Connectome

The connectome is a comprehensive map of neural connections in the brain. Understanding the connectome is crucial for comprehending how different brain parts interact to produce cognitive functions and behaviors.

By familiarizing ourselves with these critical concepts and terms, we lay a strong foundation for deeper exploration into the fascinating workings of the human brain and its relation to cognitive processes. These terms serve as the vocabulary of cognitive neuroscience and as building blocks for constructing a more nuanced understanding of how our brains enable us to perceive, think, and interact with the world around us.

1.3 The Structure and Function of the Nervous System

The nervous system is an intricate network that orchestrates a vast range of physiological and cognitive functions, serving as the command center for the entire body. It is divided into two main parts: the central nervous system (CNS) and the peripheral nervous system (PNS). Understanding the structure and function of these components is crucial for delving into the complexities of cognitive neuroscience and neuropsychology. This section provides an overview of the nervous system, highlighting its essential components and their roles.

Central Nervous System (CNS)

The CNS is comprised of the brain and spinal cord. It is the primary control center for processing and coordinating information throughout the body.

- **The Brain:** The brain is the command center for the nervous system, responsible for interpreting sensory information, generating thoughts and emotions, and coordinating movement. It is divided into several regions, each with specific functions:

  - The **cerebral cortex** is the outer layer of the brain, involved in high-level functions such as reasoning, language, and consciousness. It is divided into four lobes: frontal, parietal, temporal, and occipital, each associated with different functions.

- The **limbic system**, including the hippocampus and amygdala, plays a crucial role in emotion and memory.

  - The **basal ganglia** are involved in movement control and decision-making.

  - The **thalamus** acts as a relay station for sensory and motor signals.

  - The **hypothalamus** regulates physiological functions such as hunger, thirst, and body temperature.

- **The Spinal Cord:** The spinal cord transmits information between the brain and the rest of the body. It also coordinates reflexes and simple motor responses.

Peripheral Nervous System (PNS)

The PNS consists of all the nerves that lie outside the CNS. It is divided into the somatic nervous system and the autonomic nervous system.

- **Somatic Nervous System:** This system controls voluntary movements and conveys sensory information from the body to the CNS. It includes nerves that innervate the skin, muscles, and joints.

- **Autonomic Nervous System (ANS):** The ANS regulates involuntary bodily functions, such as heart rate, digestion, and respiratory rate. It is further divided into the sympathetic and parasympathetic nervous systems:

  - The **sympathetic nervous system** prepares the body for stress-related activities, often called the "fight or flight" response.

- The **parasympathetic nervous system** conserves energy by slowing down the heart rate and increasing intestinal and gland activity, sometimes called the "rest and digest" response.

Functional Specialization and Integration

One of the remarkable features of the nervous system is its ability to specialize and integrate functions. Different parts of the CNS and PNS are specialized for particular tasks, such as vision, hearing, movement, and emotion. However, these systems do not operate in isolation. Integration allows for the coordinated activity that underlies complex behaviors and cognitive processes. Neural pathways connect disparate brain and nervous system regions, facilitating communication and the seamless execution of functions.

The Dynamic Nervous System

Neuroplasticity is a defining characteristic of the nervous system, allowing it to change and adapt in response to experience, learning, and injury. This adaptability is evident in rewiring neural circuits throughout life and is a focal point of research in cognitive neuroscience and neuropsychology.

By understanding the structure and function of the nervous system, we gain insights into the biological foundations of behavior, thought, and emotion. This knowledge is crucial for unraveling the complexities of the human mind and forms the cornerstone of our exploration into cognitive neuroscience and neuropsychology.

1.4 Exercise: 10 MCQs with Answers at the End

Test your understanding of the foundational concepts of cognitive neuroscience with the following multiple-choice questions (MCQs). Answers are provided at the end of this section to help you assess your comprehension.

1. What is the basic unit of the nervous system?

   - A) Synapse

   - B) Neuron

   - C) Neurotransmitter

   - D) Glial cell

2. Which part of the neuron is responsible for transmitting information to other neurons?

   - A) Dendrite

   - B) Axon

   - C) Soma

   - D) Myelin sheath

3. Which of the following is NOT a cerebral cortex function?

   - A) Processing visual information

   - B) Regulating autonomic functions

   - C) Language comprehension

   - D) Decision making

4. Neuroplasticity refers to:

   - A) The brain's capacity to form new neural connections.

   - B) A neurotransmitter's ability to change its function.

   - C) The number of neurons in the brain.

   - D) The plastic nature of the brain's outer layer.

5. The limbic system plays a crucial role in:

   - A) Movement coordination.

   - B) Sensory relay.

   - C) Emotion and memory.

   - D) Visual processing.

6. Hemispheric lateralization refers to:

   - A) The division of the brain into two hemispheres.

   - B) The specialization of specific functions in one brain hemisphere.

- C) The lateral movement of hemispheres during cognitive tasks.

- D) The equal distribution of cognitive functions across both hemispheres.

7. Which imaging technique measures brain activity by detecting changes associated with blood flow?

- A) EEG

- B) MRI

- C) fMRI

- D) PET

8. The autonomic nervous system is responsible for controlling:

- A) Voluntary movements.

- B) Involuntary bodily functions.

- C) Memory formation.

- D) Language production.

9. Which neurotransmitter is primarily involved in mood regulation?

- A) Dopamine

- B) Serotonin

- C) Acetylcholine

- D) Glutamate

10. What is the role of the myelin sheath?

   - A) To relay sensory information to the brain.

   - B) To protect and insulate axons.

   - C) To produce neurotransmitters.

   - D) To regulate the speed of neural transmission.

Answers:

1. B) Neuron

2. B) Axon

3. B) Regulating autonomic functions

4. A) The brain's capacity to form new neural connections.

5. C) Emotion and memory.

6. B) The specialization of specific functions in one brain hemisphere.

7. C) fMRI

8. B) Involuntary bodily functions.

9. B) Serotonin

10. B) To protect and insulate axons.

This exercise reinforces your understanding of cognitive neuroscience's core principles and structures. Reviewing these questions and their answers lets you gauge your grasp of the subject matter and identify areas that may require further study or clarification.

Chapter 2: Neural Communication

2.1 Neurons and How They Communicate

Neural communication is the cornerstone of all cognitive and physiological functions, enabling the complex thinking, feeling, and acting processes. Neurons orchestrate this intricate information exchange system, the specialized cells that transmit signals throughout the nervous system. Understanding how neurons communicate is fundamental to grasping the principles of cognitive neuroscience and neuropsychology.

The Structure of Neurons

Neurons have a unique structure that facilitates their communication role:

- **Cell Body (Soma):** Contains the nucleus and is the metabolic center of the neuron, responsible for maintaining the cell's health.

- **Dendrites:** Branch-like structures that receive messages from other neurons and convey them toward the cell body.

- **Axon:** A long, thin fiber that transmits signals away from the cell body to other neurons, muscles, or glands. Axons can be wrapped in a myelin sheath, which accelerates signal transmission.

- **Synaptic Terminals:** The endpoints of the axon, which release neurotransmitters into the synapse, the gap between neurons.

The Process of Neural Communication

Neural communication involves the transmission of electrical and chemical signals in a multi-step process:

1. **Resting Potential:** Neurons have a resting membrane potential, with the inside of the neuron being negatively charged relative to the outside. This polarization is maintained by ion channels and pumps in the neuron's membrane.

2. **Action Potential:** When a neuron receives a sufficient signal from its dendrites, it triggers an action potential, a rapid membrane potential reversal. This electrical impulse travels along the axon to the synaptic terminals.

3. **Synaptic Transmission:** Upon reaching the synaptic terminals, the action potential causes the release of neurotransmitters, chemical messengers that cross the synaptic gap.

4. **Receptor Binding:** Neurotransmitters bind to specific receptors on the receiving neuron's dendrites, generating a new signal within it. Depending on the type of neurotransmitter and receptor, this signal can either excite or inhibit the neuron, promoting or preventing the generation of a new action potential.

5. **Signal Propagation:** If the signal is strong enough to reach the receiving neuron's threshold, it will trigger an action potential, continuing the communication process.

6. **Termination:** Neurotransmitter activity is terminated through reuptake (neurotransmitters are taken back into the sending neuron), degradation (enzymes break down the neurotransmitters), or diffusion (neurotransmitters move out of the synaptic gap).

Types of Neural Communication

- **Excitatory Transmission:** Increases the likelihood that the receiving neuron will fire an action potential, typically involving neurotransmitters like glutamate.

- **Inhibitory Transmission:** Decreases the likelihood that the receiving neuron will fire, often involving neurotransmitters such as GABA.

The Importance of Synaptic Plasticity

Synaptic plasticity, the ability of synapses to strengthen or weaken over time, is essential for learning and memory. It is based on the principle of "use it or lose it," where frequently used connections become more robust, and those rarely used weaken and may eventually disappear.

Neural communication is a dynamic and complex process that allows the nervous system to function cohesively. By understanding how neurons communicate, we gain insights into the fundamental mechanisms that underlie all cognitive functions and behaviors, paving the way for advances in treating neurological and psychiatric disorders.

2.2 Neurotransmitters and Their Roles

Neurotransmitters are the nervous system's chemical messengers, playing a pivotal role in neural communication by transmitting signals across synapses from one neuron to another. Their actions are crucial for everything from essential bodily functions to complex cognitive processes. This section explores the diverse roles of neurotransmitters and how they influence brain function and behavior.

Types of Neurotransmitters

Neurotransmitters can be broadly classified into several categories based on their functions and effects on the receiving neuron:

- **Excitatory Neurotransmitters:** Promote the firing of action potentials by increasing the likelihood that a neuron will send a signal. **Glutamate** is the most abundant excitatory neurotransmitter in the vertebrate nervous system, playing a pivotal role in synaptic plasticity and neural communication.

- **Inhibitory Neurotransmitters:** Prevent action potentials, reducing neuronal activity. **Gamma-aminobutyric acid (GABA)** is the primary inhibitory neurotransmitter in the brain, crucial for regulating neuronal excitability and preventing overstimulation.

- **Modulatory Neurotransmitters:** Have more diffuse effects, often influencing many neurons simultaneously. **Serotonin** and **dopamine** are examples of affecting mood, sleep, and motivation, among other functions.

Key Neurotransmitters and Their Functions

- **Dopamine:** Associated with the brain's reward system, dopamine plays a critical role in motivation, pleasure, and motor control. Imbalances in dopamine levels have been linked to disorders such as Parkinson's disease (low levels) and schizophrenia (high levels).

- **Serotonin:** Influences mood, appetite, sleep, memory, and learning. Low levels of serotonin are associated with depression and anxiety disorders.

- **Acetylcholine:** Involved in muscle activation, attention, memory, and learning. Dysregulation of acetylcholine is evident in Alzheimer's disease, characterized by memory loss and cognitive decline.

- **Norepinephrine:** Acts as a neurotransmitter and a hormone, playing a vital role in the body's fight or flight response. It affects attention, perception, and arousal.

- **Glutamate:** The primary excitatory neurotransmitter in the brain, glutamate is essential for cognitive functions such as learning and memory

. Its imbalance is implicated in neurological disorders like epilepsy (excessive excitation) and certain neurodegenerative diseases.

- **GABA (Gamma-Aminobutyric Acid):** As the primary inhibitory neurotransmitter, GABA helps to balance neuronal activity, preventing excessive firing that could lead to anxiety, seizures, and other conditions.

Neurotransmitter Systems and Their Impact on Behavior

Neurotransmitter systems refer to the groups of neurons that communicate using the same neurotransmitter. These systems span different brain regions and play integral roles in regulating various behaviors and physiological processes. For example:

- The **dopaminergic system** influences reward, motivation, and fine motor control. Dysfunctions in this system are linked to addiction, depression, and Parkinson's disease.

- The **serotonergic system** regulates mood, anxiety, and sleep cycles. Alterations in serotonin levels or receptor function are associated with depression, anxiety disorders, and schizophrenia.

- The **cholinergic system** (utilizing acetylcholine) is essential for memory and learning. Degeneration of cholinergic neurons in the brain is a hallmark of Alzheimer's disease.

Mechanisms of Neurotransmitter Action

Neurotransmitters exert their effects by binding to specific receptors on the post-synaptic neuron. These receptors can be ionotropic, directly opening ion channels and rapidly changing the neuron's membrane potential, or metabotropic, indirectly influencing neuronal activity through G-proteins and second messengers, leading to longer-lasting effects.

Neurotransmitters and Neuropsychology

Understanding the roles of neurotransmitters is crucial in neuropsychology, as it helps explain the biochemical underpinnings of cognition, emotion, and behavior. This knowledge is instrumental in developing pharmacological treatments for mental health disorders, aiming to correct imbalances in neurotransmitter systems. For example, selective serotonin reuptake inhibitors (SSRIs) are used to treat depression by increasing serotonin levels in the brain, demonstrating the direct application of neurotransmitter research in clinical settings.

In summary, neurotransmitters are essential for properly functioning the nervous system, influencing a broad spectrum of physiological and psychological processes. Their study provides valuable insights into the mechanisms of neural communication, the basis of behavior, and the pathophysiology of various neurological and psychiatric disorders, highlighting their significance in cognitive neuroscience and neuropsychology.

2.3 Synaptic Plasticity and Learning

Synaptic plasticity is the ability of synapses, the connections between neurons, to strengthen or weaken over time in response to increases or decreases in their activity. This adaptability is a fundamental mechanism underlying learning and memory in the brain. Through synaptic plasticity, experiences can lead to changes in synaptic efficiency, thereby modifying the strength of neural circuits and influencing behavior. This section delves into the relationship between synaptic plasticity and learning, highlighting key concepts and mechanisms.

Hebbian Plasticity: The Basis of Learning and Memory

In his seminal work, Donald Hebb proposed that "neurons that fire together, wire together." This principle, known as Hebbian plasticity, suggests that the simultaneous activation of neurons leads to pronounced increases in synaptic strength between those cells. This concept forms the basis of associative learning, where the association between two stimuli becomes stronger through repeated exposure.

Long-Term Potentiation (LTP) and Long-Term Depression (LTD)

Two primary mechanisms of synaptic plasticity are long-term potentiation (LTP) and long-term depression (LTD):

- **LTP** is an increase in synaptic strength following high-frequency stimulation of a synapse. It is considered a central cellular mechanism underlying learning and memory. LTP enhances the synaptic response to subsequent stimuli, facilitating more efficient neural communication.

- **LTD**, conversely, is a long-lasting decrease in synaptic strength resulting from the low-frequency stimulation of a synapse. LTD is thought to play a role in forgetting or the selective pruning of unnecessary synaptic connections, which is crucial for cognitive flexibility and the optimization of neural networks.

Mechanisms Underpinning Synaptic Plasticity

Synaptic plasticity involves complex molecular and cellular mechanisms:

- **Alterations in Neurotransmitter Release:** Changes in the probability of neurotransmitter release from the presynaptic neuron can enhance or reduce synaptic efficacy.

- **Receptor Trafficking:** The addition or removal of receptors, particularly glutamate receptors such as AMPA receptors, on the postsynaptic membrane can increase or decrease synaptic strength, respectively.

- **Structural Changes:** Synaptic plasticity can also lead to morphological changes, such as the growth of new dendritic spines (small protrusions on dendrites where synapses are located) or the retraction of existing ones, altering the connectivity between neurons.

The Role of Synaptic Plasticity in Learning and Memory

Synaptic plasticity is crucial for the brain's ability to encode, store, and retrieve information. For example:

- **Skill Learning:** Repeated practice of a skill leads to the strengthening of synaptic connections within relevant neural circuits, making the execution of the skill more efficient and automatic.

- **Associative Learning:** Experiences that involve associating one stimulus with another modify synaptic strength in ways that encode this relationship, allowing for the recall of associations.

- **Spatial Learning:** Navigation and spatial memory involve changes in synaptic connections within the hippocampus, demonstrating the role of plasticity in encoding information about the environment.

Implications for Neuropsychology and Education

Understanding synaptic plasticity has profound implications for neuropsychology and education. It highlights the brain's capacity for change and adaptation, suggesting that cognitive abilities can be enhanced through targeted interventions and learning experiences. Additionally, it provides insights into the pathophysiology of neurological and psychiatric disorders characterized by abnormal synaptic plasticity, guiding the development of therapeutic strategies.

In summary, synaptic plasticity is a dynamic process that plays a crucial role in learning and memory. By enabling the modification of synaptic strength in response to activity, it allows the brain to adapt to new information, experiences, and environments, highlighting the inherent adaptability of the nervous system.

2.4 Exercise: 10 MCQs with Answers at the End

Evaluate your understanding of neural communication, including the roles of neurotransmitters and synaptic plasticity in learning, with the following multiple-choice questions. Answers are provided at the end for self-assessment.

1. What type of signal is primarily used by neurons to communicate across a synapse?

   - A) Kinetic

   - B) Chemical

   - C) Thermal

- D) Optical

2. Which neurotransmitter is most commonly associated with excitatory signals in the brain?

   - A) GABA

   - B) Dopamine

   - C) Glutamate

   - D) Serotonin

3. Long-Term Potentiation (LTP) is:

   - A) A decrease in synaptic strength.

   - B) An increase in synaptic strength.

   - C) Unrelated to synaptic activity.

   - D) A temporary synaptic effect.

4. Which mechanism does NOT contribute to synaptic plasticity?

   - A) Alterations in neurotransmitter release.

   - B) Movement of ions across the synaptic cleft.

   - C) Receptor trafficking on the postsynaptic membrane.

   - D) Structural changes in synaptic connections.

5. The principle that "neurons that fire together, wire together" is known as:

- A) Pavlovian theory.

- B) Hebbian theory.

- C) Newtonian theory.

- D) Darwinian theory.

6. What role does serotonin play in the nervous system?

- A) It primarily inhibits neural activity.

- B) It modulates mood, appetite, and sleep.

- C) It excites cardiovascular function.

- D) It decreases memory and learning capabilities.

7. Which of the following is a characteristic feature of Long-Term Depression (LTD)?

- A) It enhances memory retention.

- B) It increases the efficiency of synaptic transmission.

- C) It involves the removal of AMPA receptors from the postsynaptic membrane.

- D) It is triggered by high-frequency stimulation of a synapse.

8. Synaptic plasticity is essential for:

   - A) Only memory formation.

   - B) Only cognitive flexibility.

   - C) Both learning and memory.

   - D) Only sensory perception.

9. The process by which neurotransmitters are taken back into the presynaptic neuron is called:

   - A) Reuptake.

   - B) Degradation.

   - C) Diffusion.

   - D) Exocytosis.

10. Acetylcholine is involved in:

   - A) Only muscle activation.

   - B) Only attention and arousal.

   - C) Memory, learning, and muscle activation.

   - D) Only the regulation of mood.

Answers:

1. B) Chemical

2. C) Glutamate

3. B) An increase in synaptic strength.

4. B) Movement of ions across the synaptic cleft.

5. B) Hebbian theory.

6. B) It modulates mood, appetite, and sleep.

7. C) It involves the removal of AMPA receptors from the postsynaptic membrane.

8. C) Both learning and memory.

9. A) Reuptake.

10. C) Memory, learning, and muscle activation.

These questions are designed to test your knowledge of the fundamental principles of neural communication, the role of neurotransmitters, and the importance of synaptic plasticity in learning and memory. By reviewing your answers, you can assess your understanding of these complex processes and identify areas for further study.

Chapter 3: Sensation and Perception

3.1 The Visual System

The visual system is a complex network that transforms light into a coherent representation of the world around us, enabling us to navigate our environment, recognize faces, and appreciate beauty. This intricate process involves multiple stages, from the initial detection of light by the eyes to the interpretation of visual information by the brain. Understanding the optical system sheds light on how we see and how the brain processes information to create our perception of reality.

Anatomy of the Eye

The eye functions like a camera, capturing light and converting it into electrical signals the brain can process. Key components include:

- **Cornea:** The clear, dome-shaped surface that covers the front of the eye, helping to focus incoming light.

- **Lens:** Located behind the iris, the lens focuses light on the retina. Its shape can change to adjust focus, a process known as accommodation.

- **Retina:** The light-sensitive layer of tissue at the back of the eye, containing photoreceptor cells (rods and cones) that detect light and color.

- **Rods:** Specialized for low-light conditions and peripheral vision, rods are susceptible to brightness but do not distinguish colors.

- **Cones:** Cones are responsible for color vision and detail in well-lit conditions. Cones are concentrated in the fovea, the center of the retina's visual field.

From Light to Electrical Signals

When light reaches the retina, it triggers a chemical reaction in the photoreceptor cells, converting the light into electrical signals. These signals are then processed by other retinal cells (bipolar cells, ganglion cells) before being transmitted to the brain through the optic nerve.

Visual Pathways to the Brain

The journey from the eyes to the brain involves several key steps:

- **Optic Nerve:** Carries visual information from the retina to the optic chiasm, where fibers from the nasal (inner) halves of each retina cross to the opposite side of the brain.

- **Optic Tracts:** After the optic chiasm, the fibers continue as optic tracts, carrying information to various brain parts, including the thalamus and the superior colliculus.

- **Lateral Geniculate Nucleus (LGN) of the Thalamus:** Acts as a relay station, sending visual information to the occipital lobe's primary visual cortex (V1).

- **Primary Visual Cortex and Beyond** In V1, the visual information is processed further and distributed to secondary visible areas (V2, V3, V4, etc.) for more complex processing involving shape, color, motion, and depth perception.

Visual Processing: Beyond the Primary Visual Cortex

Visual processing involves two main pathways, often referred to as the "what" and "where" pathways:

- **The Ventral Stream (What Pathway):** Extends from the primary visual cortex to the temporal lobe, involved in object recognition and form representation.

- **The Dorsal Stream (Where Pathway):** Projects from the primary visual cortex to the parietal lobe involve spatial awareness and movement.

The Visual System and Perception

Perception is not merely a passive reflection of the external world but an active process of interpretation. To construct a coherent world representation, the brain integrates visual information with past experiences, expectations, and contextual cues. This explains why perception can vary among individuals and in different conditions, highlighting the subjective nature of our visual experience.

In summary, the visual system is a testament to the complexity and efficiency of neural processing, converting light into meaningful perceptions that guide our interactions with the environment. Understanding this system provides insights into the biological basis of vision and the nature of perception itself, revealing the intricate interplay between sensory input and cognitive processes.

3.2 Auditory Processing

Auditory processing is the complex sequence of steps by which sound waves in the environment are transformed into meaningful auditory experiences. This process involves detecting, analyzing, and interpreting sound, engaging various structures of the ear and brain to decode sound waves into a form that can be understood and responded to. Here, we explore the journey of sound from its source to our cognitive recognition.

Anatomy of the Ear

The ear is divided into three main parts: the outer ear, the middle ear, and the inner ear, each playing a crucial role in hearing.

- **Outer Ear:** Comprises the pinna (the visible part of the ear) and the ear canal. The outer ear captures sound waves and funnels them toward the eardrum.

- **Middle Ear:** Contains three tiny bones called the ossicles (malleus, incus, and stapes), which amplify the vibrations from the eardrum and transmit them to the inner ear.

- **Inner Ear:** Houses the cochlea, a spiral-shaped, fluid-filled organ that converts sound vibrations into electrical signals. The cochlea contains tiny hair cells that move in response to fluid vibrations, triggering neural signals.

From Sound Waves to Neural Signals

The transformation of sound into a form that the brain can recognize involves several steps:

1. **Sound Wave Capture:** Sound waves enter the ear canal, causing the eardrum to vibrate.

2. **Amplification:** The ossicles in the middle ear amplify these vibrations and transmit them to the cochlea's oval window.

3. **Cochlear Processing:** Vibrations cause the fluid inside the cochlea to move, bending the hair cells. This movement generates electrical signals by altering the permeability of the hair cell membranes to ions.

4. **Auditory Nerve:** The electrical signals activate the auditory nerve fibers, which carry the acoustic information to the brain.

Auditory Pathways to the Brain

Once in the brain, the auditory signals follow a complex pathway to be processed:

- **Cochlear Nuclei:** The auditory nerve fibers first synapse at the brainstem's cochlear nuclei.

- **Superior Olivary Complex:** Signals are then relayed to the superior olivary complex, where cues for sound localization are processed.

- **Inferior Colliculus:** The pathway continues to the inferior colliculus, a vital relay station in the midbrain that integrates auditory input with other sensory information.

- **Medial Geniculate Body (MGB) of the Thalamus:** Auditory signals are further processed in the MGB, a relay to the primary auditory cortex.

- **Primary Auditory Cortex:** Located in the temporal lobe, this is where the conscious perception of sound begins. Different areas of the auditory cortex are specialized for processing various aspects of sound, such as frequency, intensity, and temporal patterns.

Understanding and Interpreting Sounds

The brain interprets the signals from the auditory cortex to recognize speech, music, environmental sounds, and their spatial locations. This involves both the primary auditory cortex and higher-level auditory areas that analyze the complex features of sound, enabling us to understand language, appreciate music, and navigate our environment using auditory cues.

The Role of Auditory Plasticity

Auditory processing is also subject to plasticity, allowing the brain to adapt to changes in auditory input. This plasticity is essential for developing language skills in children and can be observed in adults learning new languages or adjusting to hearing loss.

In summary, auditory processing is a multifaceted process that converts sound waves into meaningful auditory experiences. This process exemplifies the brain's remarkable ability to interpret complex sensory information, enabling us to communicate, enjoy music, and remain alert to our surroundings.

3.3 Touch, Taste, and Smell

The sensory systems of touch, taste, and smell provide critical information about our environment, enabling us to interact meaningfully with the world. Though less often spotlighted than vision and hearing, these systems play vital roles in our survival, communication, and enjoyment of life. This section delves into the mechanisms of touch, taste, and smell, revealing how these senses process and interpret stimuli.

Touch: The Somatosensory System

The sense of touch, or tactile sensation, involves detecting physical pressure, temperature, and pain. It is mediated by the somatosensory system, distributed throughout the body in the skin, muscles, and internal organs.

- **Mechanoreceptors:** Specialized nerve endings in the skin respond to mechanical stimuli such as pressure, vibration, and stretch. Mechanoreceptors are tuned to other touch sensations, including Merkel cells, Meissner's corpuscles, Ruffini endings, and Pacinian corpuscles.

- **Thermoreceptors:** Detect temperature changes with distinct receptors for warm and cold sensations.

- **Nociceptors:** Respond to potentially damaging stimuli by sending signals that are perceived as pain to the brain.

Touch information is relayed from the peripheral nervous system to the central nervous system, which is processed in the brain's somatosensory cortex. This processing allows us to determine tactile stimuli's location, intensity, and quality.

Taste: The Gustatory System

Taste, or gustation, enables us to detect and differentiate the flavors of substances. The gustatory system is primarily located in the taste buds on the tongue, which are sensitive to five basic tastes: sweet, sour, salty, bitter, and umami (savory).

- **Taste Buds:** Each taste bud contains taste receptor cells that respond to specific chemicals in food. When these chemicals bind to receptors, they trigger electrical signals sent to the brain.

- **Gustatory Pathways:** Taste signals are carried to the brainstem and then to the thalamus, which relays them to the gustatory cortex in the brain. Here, taste sensations are integrated with smell and other sensory information to produce the overall flavor of food.

Smell: The Olfactory System

Smell, or olfaction, is the detection of airborne chemicals by the olfactory system. It is a direct and consequential sense, capable of triggering memories and emotions.

- **Olfactory Receptors:** Located in the olfactory epithelium in the upper part of the nasal cavity, olfactory receptors recognize specific molecules in the air. Humans have approximately 400 types of olfactory receptors, allowing us to detect a wide range of smells.

- **Olfactory Bulb:** Olfactory receptor neurons send signals to the olfactory bulb, a structure at the base of the brain. From here, olfactory information is sent to various brain regions, including the olfactory cortex, the amygdala, and the hippocampus, which are involved in smell identification, emotional response, and memory.

Integration of Sensory Information

Touch, taste, and smell interact closely with each other and with other sensory systems to create our perception of the world. For example, the flavor of food is a combination of taste and smell, and the texture of an object can influence how its weight is perceived. This multisensory integration is crucial for accurately interpreting our environment and responding appropriately.

In summary, the senses of touch, taste, and smell each utilize unique mechanisms to convert physical or chemical stimuli into neural signals that the brain can interpret. These senses enrich our interactions with the world, influencing our preferences, behaviors, and memories.

3.4 Exercise: 10 MCQs with Answers at the End

Test your understanding of the sensory systems of touch, taste, and smell with these multiple-choice questions. Answers are provided at the end for self-assessment.

1. Which type of receptor is responsible for detecting temperature changes?

   - A) Mechanoreceptors

   - B) Thermoreceptors

   - C) Nociceptors

   - D) Olfactory receptors

2. The sense of taste is also known as:

   - A) Olfaction

   - B) Gustation

   - C) Audition

   - D) Proprioception

3. What is the primary role of Meissner's corpuscles?

   - A) Detecting pressure

   - B) Sensing temperature

- C) Perceiving delicate touch and texture

- D) Responding to pain

4. Which basic taste is associated with the flavor enhancer monosodium glutamate (MSG)?

- A) Sweet

- B) Sour

- C) Umami

- D) Bitter

5. Where are olfactory receptors located?

- A) In the taste buds

- B) On the skin

- C) In the olfactory epithelium of the nasal cavity

- D) In the auditory canal

6. Pacinian corpuscles are highly sensitive to:

- A) Light touch

- B) Vibration and deep pressure

- C) Changes in temperature

- D) Chemical stimuli

7. Which part of the brain is primarily involved in taste perception?

   - A) The somatosensory cortex

   - B) The gustatory cortex

   - C) The olfactory bulb

   - D) The auditory cortex

8. The combination of smell and taste contributes to:

   - A) The vestibular sense

   - B) The perception of flavor

   - C) The detection of pain

   - D) The sense of balance

9. Nociceptors are specialized receptors that detect:

   - A) Motion

   - B) Sound waves

   - C) Potentially damaging stimuli (pain)

   - D) Light

10. Umami taste receptors respond to the presence of:

   - A) Sodium ions

   - B) Sugar molecules

   - C) Glutamate

- D) Acidic substances

Answers:

1. B) Thermoreceptors

2. B) Gustation

3. C) Perceiving delicate touch and texture

4. C) Umami

5. C) In the olfactory epithelium of the nasal cavity

6. B) Vibration and deep pressure

7. B) The gustatory cortex

8. B) The perception of flavor

9. C) Potentially damaging stimuli (pain)

10. C) Glutamate

These questions reinforce your understanding of how the sensory systems of touch, taste, and smell function and interact to create our perception of the world. Reviewing these answers will help you assess your knowledge and identify areas requiring further study.

Chapter 4: Memory

4.1 Types of Memory

Memory is fundamental to human cognition and essential for learning, reasoning, and adaptation. It encompasses the processes involved in encoding, storing, and retrieving information. Over the years, research has elucidated that memory is not a single entity but a complex system composed of different types. Understanding these types helps us appreciate the breadth of human memory capabilities and the underlying mechanisms.

Sensory Memory

Sensory memory is the earliest stage of memory, which holds an exact copy of incoming sensory information for a very brief period. It acts as a buffer for stimuli received through the senses, allowing them to be noticed momentarily.

- **Iconic Memory:** Refers to the visual sensory memory, which retains an image of what you have seen for less than a second.

- **Echoic Memory:** The auditory sensory memory, holding onto sounds for 3-4 seconds, enabling you to process auditory information as a continuous stream.

Short-Term Memory (STM) / Working Memory

Short-term memory, often used interchangeably with working memory, is the capacity to hold a small amount of information in an active, readily available state for a short period. It serves as a workspace for the mind, where data is manipulated, discarded, or transferred to long-term memory.

- **Capacity:** Traditionally described as able to hold 7 ± 2 items, recent research suggests this capacity might be more limited.

- **Duration:** Information in STM lasts about 20 to 30 seconds unless actively rehearsed.

- **Working Memory:** A more complex model with several components to store and manipulate visual, spatial, and verbal information.

Long-Term Memory (LTM)

Long-term memory is the phase of memory where information is stored more permanently, potentially for a lifetime. It has a vast capacity and is categorized into explicit (declarative) and implicit (non-declarative) memory.

- **Explicit Memory:** Involves conscious recall of facts and events. It is further divided into:

  - **Episodic Memory:** For personal experiences and specific events.

- **Semantic Memory:** For general knowledge, concepts, facts, and meanings.

- **Implicit Memory:** Includes memory for skills, procedures, and conditioned responses that do not require conscious thought. It encompasses:

  - **Procedural Memory:** For skills and tasks (e.g., bike riding).

  - **Priming:** Subtle influences of past experiences on response to a stimulus.

  - **Classical Conditioning:** Learning through association, where a neutral stimulus becomes associated with a meaningful stimulus, eliciting a response.

Autobiographical Memory

A particular category of memory that contains information about ourselves and our personal history: it blends episodic and semantic memory, contributing to personal identity.

Emotional Memory

The aspect of memory that involves the emotional charge associated with a memory. It is believed that emotional experiences are better remembered than non-emotional ones, a phenomenon linked to the amygdala's role in processing emotions.

Understanding the different types of memory illuminates the complexity of the human memory system, highlighting its role in every aspect of our daily lives. From the fleeting capture of sensory details to the deep storage of personal experiences and skills, memory enables us to learn from the past, navigate the present, and plan for the future.

4.2 The Process of Memory Formation

Memory formation is a dynamic and multifaceted process that allows individuals to encode, store, and retrieve information. This process is crucial for learning, adaptation, and survival. Understanding how memories are formed involves examining the stages through which information passes from initial perception to long-term storage.

Encoding

Encoding is the first step in creating a memory. It involves transforming incoming information into a neural code the brain can use. This stage determines what information is noticed and how it is perceived. Encoding can be enhanced through attention, rehearsal, and mnemonic devices. The nature of encoding varies depending on the type of information:

- **Semantic Encoding:** Relates to encoding meaning, including understanding and applying logical structures to the information.

- **Acoustic Encoding:** Involves the encoding of sounds, particularly the sound of words.

- **Visual Encoding:** Pertains to encoding images and visual sensory information.

Consolidation

Consolidation is the process by which encoded information becomes stored in a more permanent form. It involves strengthening the neural connections that represent the memory, making it more stable and less susceptible to disruption. Two types of consolidation are recognized:

- **Synaptic Consolidation:** Occurs over hours after learning and involves changes at the synapses between neurons.

- **Systems Consolidation:** A more protracted process that can take weeks, months, or even years, where memories become integrated into the network of long-term memories stored throughout the brain.

Neuroscientific research suggests that the hippocampus plays a critical role in this process, particularly in consolidating explicit memories. During sleep, the hippocampus is believed to replay the day's events, which helps to strengthen neural connections and facilitate memory consolidation.

Storage

Storage refers to how information is retained over time. Memory is stored across different regions of the brain, depending on the memory type:

- **Sensory Memories:** Stored in the sensory area of the cortex where the information was first processed.

- **Short-Term Memories:** Primarily managed by the prefrontal cortex.

- **Long-Term Memories:** Distributed across various cortical regions; for example, the hippocampus is crucial for storing explicit memories, while the cerebellum and basal ganglia are involved in storing implicit memories.

Retrieval

Retrieval is the process of accessing and bringing the information stored in memory into consciousness. It can be influenced by various factors, including cues, context, and the specific neural pathways involved in encoding the memory. Retrieval can be a straightforward recall of facts or a more complex reconstruction of events and experiences. The success of retrieval often depends on the similarity between the encoding and retrieval environments, a phenomenon known as context-dependent memory.

Forgetting and Memory Decay

Forgetting is a normal part of the memory process, often resulting from the failure of memory retrieval. Theories of forgetting include memory decay, interference (where other memories compete), and retrieval failure due to insufficient cues or encoding specificity.

Understanding the process of memory formation provides insights into the complexities of human cognition and the underlying neural mechanisms. It also highlights the importance of various factors, such as attention, rehearsal, and emotional significance, in enhancing memory formation and retrieval.

4.3 Memory Retrieval and Forgetting

Memory retrieval and forgetting are essential aspects of the memory process, balancing the cognitive system by enabling access to stored information while managing the limitations of memory storage. This dynamic interplay ensures that relevant memories are accessible when needed while less pertinent information fades away, maintaining an efficient cognitive system.

Memory Retrieval

Memory retrieval is the process of accessing and bringing the information stored in memory into conscious thought. This process can vary in difficulty, depending on several factors, including the type of memory, the cues available, and the context of retrieval.

- **Recall:** This form of retrieval requires information retrieval without explicit cues. It is often more challenging and used in situations like essay tests.

- **Recognition:** In contrast, recognition involves identifying information in the presence of cues, such as in multiple-choice tests. It is generally easier than recall because the cues facilitate the retrieval process.

- **Relearning:** This method indicates the ease with which information can be learned or memorized after being forgotten. It often requires less effort than the initial learning, suggesting some residual memory effect.

Context-Dependent Memory

The context in which information is encoded and retrieved can significantly affect memory retrieval. Context-dependent memory is the phenomenon where recall is more effective when the retrieval context matches the encoding context. This effect underscores the importance of environmental and situational cues in memory retrieval processes.

State-Dependent Memory

Like context-dependent memory, state-dependent memory refers to the principle that memory retrieval is more efficient when an individual's internal state at retrieval matches their state during encoding. This includes emotional state, physiological state, or mood, suggesting that internal cues can also facilitate memory retrieval.

Forgetting

Forgetting is a natural and often beneficial part of the memory process, allowing the brain to prioritize relevant information and discard what is no longer needed. Several theories explain the mechanisms behind forgetting:

- **Decay Theory:** Suggests that memory traces weaken over time if not accessed or used, leading to forgetting.

- **Interference Theory:** Proposes that forgetting occurs because some memories compete and interfere. This can be:

  - **Proactive Interference:** Where old information interferes with the recall of new information.

  - **Retroactive Interference:** Where new information impacts the recall of old information.

- **Motivated Forgetting:** Based on the idea that some memories are forgotten because they are distressing or not beneficial to remember. This includes repression, a defense mechanism proposed by Freud, where traumatic memories are pushed into the unconscious.

Retrieval Failure

Retrieval failure is another explanation for forgetting, suggesting that memories are not lost but are momentarily inaccessible. The tip-of-the-tongue phenomenon is a typical example where individuals cannot retrieve information but feel on the verge of remembering it.

Improving Memory Retrieval

Strategies to improve memory retrieval include practicing effective encoding strategies, using mnemonic devices, creating associations between new information and existing knowledge, and ensuring a match between the encoding and retrieval contexts.

Understanding memory retrieval and forgetting is crucial for comprehending how memories are accessed and why some memories fade over time. It highlights the complex nature of memory as a dynamic system that not only stores information but manages it in a way that supports efficient cognitive functioning.

4.4 Exercise: 10 MCQs with Answers at the End

Evaluate your understanding of memory retrieval, forgetting and the mechanisms behind them with the following multiple-choice questions. Answers are provided at the end for self-assessment.

1. What type of memory retrieval involves identifying information with cues?

   - A) Recall

   - B) Recognition

   - C) Relearning

   - D) Repression

2. The phenomenon where recall is better when the context at retrieval matches the context during encoding is known as:

   - A) State-dependent memory

   - B) Context-dependent memory

   - C) Interference theory

   - D) Decay theory

3. Which theory suggests that forgetting occurs because memories interfere with and disrupt each other?

- A) Decay theory

- B) Interference theory

- C) Motivated forgetting

- D) Retrieval failure

4. What is it called when old information interferes with the recall of new information?

- A) Retroactive interference

- B) Proactive interference

- C) Repression

- D) Suppression

5. The tip-of-the-tongue phenomenon is an example of:

- A) Decay theory

- B) Motivated forgetting

- C) Retrieval failure

- D) Retroactive interference

6. Repression is a concept. Which type of forgetting is it?

- A) Decay theory

- B) Interference theory

- C) Motivated forgetting

- D) Retrieval failure

7. State-dependent memory refers to the principle that memory retrieval is more efficient when:

- A) The external context matches the internal state at encoding.

- B) The internal state at retrieval matches the state during encoding.

- C) The information is relearned quickly.

- D) The information is recognized, not recalled.

8. Which type of memory involves the ease with which information can be memorized again after it has been forgotten?

- A) Recall

- B) Recognition

- C) Relearning

- D) Repression

9. Decay theory of forgetting posits that forgetting occurs due to:

- A) New information overshadowing old information.

- B) The passage of time leading to memory traces fading.

- C) Intentionally suppressing unwanted memories.

- D) The context of encoding and retrieval being mismatched.

10. Which memory retrieval process requires pulling information from memory without explicit cues?

   - A) Recall

   - B) Recognition

   - C) Relearning

   - D) Repression

Answers:

1. B) Recognition

2. B) Context-dependent memory

3. B) Interference theory

4. B) Proactive interference

5. C) Retrieval failure

6. C) Motivated forgetting

7. B) The internal state at retrieval matches the state during encoding.

8. C) Relearning

9. B) The passage of time leading to memory traces fading.

10. A) Recall

These questions are designed to test your knowledge of the processes involved in memory retrieval and forgetting, helping you understand the complexity of how memories are accessed, stored, and sometimes lost. Reviewing your answers will provide insight into your grasp of these concepts and identify areas for further exploration.

Chapter 5: Language and Cognition

5.1 The Structure of Language

Language is a complex, multifaceted system that communicates ideas, emotions, and information through a structured set of symbols and sounds. Understanding language structure involves dissecting its various components, from the most minor sound units to the organization of meaningful expressions and sentences. This section explores the fundamental aspects of language structure, including phonology, morphology, syntax, semantics, and pragmatics, which form the basis of linguistic competence.

Phonology

Phonology refers to the study of the sound system of a language, including the rules for combining and using sounds (phonemes) to produce meaningful words and sentences. Phonemes are the most minor units of sound that can differentiate meaning in a language. For example, the change of a single phoneme in a word can alter its entire meaning, as seen in "bat" versus "pat."

Morphology

Morphology is the branch of linguistics concerned with the structure of words. It examines how words are formed from morphemes, the slightest meaning, or grammatical function units in a language. This includes understanding the formation of new words (derivational morphology) and the creation of different word forms (inflectional morphology), such as tense, number, or case.

Syntax

Syntax is the set of rules, principles, and processes that govern the structure of sentences in a language. It involves arranging words and phrases to create meaningful sentences following a specific grammatical structure. Syntax addresses how sentences are formed, how words interact within a sentence to convey meaning and the patterns and structures that sentences follow.

Semantics

Semantics deals with the meaning of words, phrases, sentences, and texts. It explores how linguistic signs convey meaning, how meaning is constructed in language, and how listeners and speakers understand it. Semantics encompasses the study of synonyms, antonyms, homonyms, and words' connotative versus denotative meanings.

Pragmatics

Pragmatics focuses on the use of language in context and how context influences the interpretation of meaning. It examines how speakers use language to achieve specific effects and how listeners infer meaning based on the context. Pragmatics considers factors such as the speaker's intentions, the relationship between speaker and listener, and the conventions of politeness and social interaction.

The Interplay of Language Components

The structure of language is a dynamic interplay of its various components, each contributing to the richness and versatility of human communication. Phonology and morphology deal with the form of language, syntax structures, and linguistic expressions; semantics provide meaning, and pragmatics bridges language with its use in social contexts. Together, these elements define the complexity of human language, enabling nuanced and effective communication across different cultures and contexts.

Understanding language structure is essential for exploring how language influences cognitive processes, including thought, memory, and perception. It also sheds light on the development of language acquisition, language disorders, and the cognitive mechanisms underlying linguistic abilities.

5.2 Language Acquisition

Language acquisition is a fascinating process through which humans learn to communicate using the languages around them. This complex cognitive achievement involves acquiring a language's sounds, structures, and meanings, often starting from infancy. Language acquisition encompasses children's natural uptake of a first language (L1) and the learning of additional languages (L2) later in life. Understanding this process sheds light on humans' innate cognitive capabilities for language and the factors that influence linguistic development.

Stages of First Language Acquisition

First language acquisition typically unfolds through several identifiable stages, each marked by specific milestones:

- **Pre-linguistic Stage:** Before speaking, infants engage in vocal play, producing sounds like cooing and babbling. This stage is crucial for practicing the motor skills required for speech.

- **One-Word Stage:** Around the age of one, children begin to use single words to convey whole ideas, such as "milk" for wanting milk. These words often serve multiple purposes depending on context.

- **Two-Word Stage:** By age two, children start combining two words to form simple sentences, like "more cookie," demonstrating an understanding of syntactic relations.

- **Telegraphic Stage:** Children then produce "telegraphic" speech resembling a telegram. They use short sentences that contain only essential content words, omitting smaller function words and inflections, e.g., "Mommy, go store."

- **Complex Sentences:** As children's vocabulary and understanding of grammar expand, they begin constructing more complex sentences, incorporating broader vocabulary and grammatical structures.

Theories of Language Acquisition

Several theories have been proposed to explain how children acquire language:

- **Nativist Theory:** Proposed by Noam Chomsky, this theory suggests that humans are born with a language acquisition device (LAD), an innate biological capacity to learn language. According to Chomsky, universal grammar underlies all human languages, enabling children to acquire any language they are exposed to easily.

- **Social Interactionist Theory:** Emphasizes the role of social interaction in language development. It suggests that language acquisition is driven by the child's desire to communicate with others, with learning facilitated by interaction with more competent language users.

- **Cognitive Theory:** Proposes that language acquisition is part of broader cognitive development. According to this view, children's ability to learn language is tied to their overall cognitive skills and the development of mental processes such as memory, attention, and perception.

- **Connectionist Models:** Suggest that language acquisition results from strengthening neural connections in the brain. These models emphasize the importance of exposure and repetition in learning the patterns and structures of language.

Factors Influencing Language Acquisition

Language development can be influenced by a variety of factors, including:

- **Genetic Dispositions:** Individual differences in linguistic ability can be partly attributed to genetics.

- **Social Interaction:** The quantity and quality of linguistic input and interaction children receive are crucial for language development.

- **Cognitive Abilities:** General cognitive skills, including working memory and processing speed, can affect language learning.

- **Motivation and Attitude:** Particularly relevant for second language acquisition, a learner's motivation and attitude towards the language can significantly impact their success.

Understanding language acquisition provides insights into human cognitive development and informs educational practices, speech therapy, and the development of artificial intelligence systems designed to mimic human language understanding.

5.3 Cognitive Processes in Language Use

Language use is a sophisticated cognitive function that involves various mental processes. These processes enable individuals to understand, produce, and communicate complex ideas through spoken, written, and signed language modes. The cognitive underpinnings of language use encompass perception, memory, attention, and problem-solving, working together to facilitate linguistic comprehension and expression. This section explores vital cognitive processes involved in language use, including comprehension, speech production, reading, writing, and bilingualism.

Language Comprehension

Language comprehension involves decoding and understanding spoken, written, or signed language. It relies on the interaction between:

- **Phonological Processing:** The ability to recognize and manipulate the sound structures of language.

- **Syntactic Processing:** Understanding the grammatical structure of sentences to glean meaning.

- **Semantic Processing:** The interpretation of the meaning of words and sentences, integrating this information with existing knowledge.

- **Pragmatic Understanding:** Grasping the intended meaning behind language use in context, considering the speaker's intentions, social norms, and the conversational setting.

Speech Production

Speech production is a complex process that transforms thoughts into spoken words. This involves:

- **Conceptualization:** Generating an idea or message to communicate.

- **Formulation:** Selecting appropriate words and arranging them in a grammatically correct sequence.

- **Articulation:** Physically producing speech sounds through the coordinated movement of the mouth, tongue, and respiratory system.

- **Self-Monitoring:** Listening to one's speech to ensure accuracy and making real-time adjustments as needed.

Reading and Writing

Reading and writing are advanced language skills that involve additional cognitive processes:

- **Decoding:** In reading, decoding involves translating written text into sounds or directly into meanings for word recognition.

- **Lexical Access:** Quickly accessing word meanings from memory during reading and writing.

- **Comprehension:** Building meaning from text, integrating new information with existing knowledge.

- **Composition:** In writing, organizing thoughts and structuring them according to linguistic conventions to convey a message effectively.

Bilingualism and Multilingualism

Bilingualism and multilingualism introduce complexity to cognitive processes in language use. Managing multiple language systems requires:

- **Language Selection:** Choosing the appropriate language based on the context.

- **Code-Switching:** Alternating between languages within a conversation or even a sentence, requiring flexible cognitive control.

- **Cross-Linguistic Influence:** Experiencing the influence of one language on the use and understanding of another, which can affect vocabulary, syntax, and phonology.

Cognitive Benefits of Language Use

Engaging in complex language use, especially in multilingual contexts, can enhance cognitive flexibility, attentional control, and problem-solving abilities. Studies have shown that bilingualism, in particular, may contribute to a cognitive reserve that delays the onset of dementia symptoms.

Neurocognitive Foundations

Specific brain regions and networks support the cognitive processes in language use. For example, Broca's area involves speech production, while Wernicke's is crucial for language comprehension. The connection between these areas, through the arcuate fasciculus, facilitates the integration of comprehension and production processes.

In summary, the cognitive processes involved in language use are intricate and multifaceted, drawing on various aspects of human cognition. Understanding these processes illuminates the complexity of language as a human faculty. It provides insights into the cognitive benefits of language learning and use and the neurocognitive infrastructure that supports linguistic abilities.

5.4 Exercise: 10 MCQs with Answers at the End

Test your understanding of language and cognition with these multiple-choice questions. Answers are provided at the end for self-assessment.

1. Which cognitive process is primarily involved in understanding the grammatical structure of sentences?

   - A) Syntactic processing

- B) Semantic processing

- C) Phonological processing

- D) Pragmatic understanding

2. The ability to produce speech involves all the following steps EXCEPT:

- A) Conceptualization

- B) Formulation

- C) Decoding

- D) Articulation

3. What term describes the phenomenon of switching between languages within a conversation?

- A) Bilingualism

- B) Lexical access

- C) Code-switching

- D) Cross-linguistic influence

4. Which area of the brain is primarily associated with language comprehension?

- A) Broca's area

- B) Wernicke's area

- C) Amygdala

- D) Hippocampus

5. The cognitive process that allows for the quick accessing of word meanings during reading and writing is called:

- A) Decoding

- B) Lexical access

- C) Comprehension

- D) Composition

6. What is the first step in the speech production process?

- A) Formulation

- B) Conceptualization

- C) Articulation

- D) Self-Monitoring

7. Managing multiple language systems in bilingualism requires:

- A) Phonological processing

- B) Language selection

- C) Semantic processing

- D) Syntactic processing

8. The integration of new information with existing knowledge during reading is part of:

- A) Decoding

- B) Lexical access

- C) Comprehension

- D) Composition

9. Which cognitive process involves interpreting the meaning of words and sentences?

- A) Syntactic processing

- B) Semantic processing

- C) Phonological processing

- D) Pragmatic understanding

10. Cross-linguistic influence is a concept that explains:

- A) The ability to speak more than one language

- B) The influence of one language on the learning of another

- C) The process of learning a second language

- D) The switching of languages during a conversation

Answers:

1. A) Syntactic processing

2. C) Decoding

3. C) Code-switching

4. B) Wernicke's area

5. B) Lexical access

6. B) Conceptualization

7. B) Language selection

8. C) Comprehension

9. B) Semantic processing

10. B) The influence of one language on the learning of another

These questions are designed to assess your knowledge of the cognitive processes involved in language use, including how language is comprehended and produced and the intricacies of bilingualism. Reviewing your answers will help you gauge your understanding of language and cognition, highlighting areas for further study or review.

Chapter 6: Executive Functions and Control

6.1 Attention and Its Mechanisms

Attention is a cognitive process crucial for almost all aspects of daily functioning, from primary sensory perception to complex decision-making. It involves the selective concentration on a discrete aspect of information, whether subjective or environmental while ignoring other perceivable information. Attention is not just a singular process but encompasses several mechanisms and systems working together to filter, prioritize, and focus on relevant stimuli.

Types of Attention

- **Selective Attention:** The ability to focus on one specific task or stimulus while ignoring other distractions. This is akin to the "spotlight" model, where the focus can shift to highlight different aspects of the environment.

- **Sustained Attention:** Also known as vigilance, this refers to the capacity to maintain attentional focus over prolonged periods. It is critical for tasks that require continuous monitoring or performance.

- **Divided Attention:** The ability to process two or more responses or react to multiple tasks simultaneously. Cognitive resources often limit this and can lead to decreased performance in tasks.

- **Executive Attention:** Associated with regulating thoughts, emotions, and responses, especially in complex situations requiring planning, error detection, decision-making, and inhibitory control.

Mechanisms of Attention

Attention is controlled through a combination of top-down and bottom-up mechanisms:

- **Top-Down Processes:** These are voluntary and driven by cognitive processes, such as when we decide to pay attention to a conversation or a task. It involves the prefrontal cortex and is influenced by our intentions, expectations, and experience.

- **Bottom-Up Processes:** These are involuntary and stimulus-driven, such as the sudden attention drawn by a loud noise. This process is mediated by the sensory cortices and the thalamus and is influenced by the properties of the stimuli.

Neural Substrates of Attention

The neural basis of attention involves multiple brain regions and networks, including:

- **The Frontal Eye Field (FEF):** Involved in controlling visual attention and eye movements.

- **The Parietal Lobes:** Play a key role in orienting attention in space and the selection of relevant stimuli.

- **The Temporal Lobes:** Involved in selective attention to auditory stimuli.

- **The Anterior Cingulate Cortex (ACC)** Important for executive attention, conflict monitoring, and the allocation of cognitive resources.

Attentional Networks

Research has identified several neural networks critical to attentional processes:

- **The Alerting Network:** Engages the brain in preparation for incoming stimuli, involving brainstem structures and the frontal and parietal lobes.

- **The Orienting Network:** Responsible for selecting information from sensory input, directing attention to locations in space or specific features.

- **The Executive Control Network:** Manages complex cognitive processes, resolving conflicts among responses, and is heavily reliant on the functions of the prefrontal cortex.

Challenges and Disorders

Attention difficulties can significantly impact daily life and are a hallmark of several neurological and psychiatric conditions, such as Attention-Deficit/Hyperactivity Disorder (ADHD), where there is a pervasive pattern of inattention, hyperactivity, and impulsivity. Understanding attention mechanisms and their neural substrates helps diagnose and treat such conditions effectively.

In summary, attention is a multifaceted cognitive function essential for processing information from our environment and internal world. It involves selective focusing, sustained vigilance, the ability to manage multiple tasks, and the executive control of thoughts and actions, supported by complex neural networks and brain regions.

6.2 Working Memory

Working memory is a critical cognitive system that temporarily stores and manipulates the information necessary for complex cognitive tasks such as language comprehension, learning, and reasoning. This concept expands on short-term memory, highlighting not just the storage but also the manipulation of information.

Components of Working Memory

The model of working memory, most notably proposed by Baddeley and Hitch (1974), outlines several components:

- **The Central Executive:** Acts as a control system that directs attention and coordinates information from the other components of working memory. It regulates the flow of information, managing cognitive tasks such as problem-solving and decision-making.

- **The Phonological Loop:** Responsible for temporarily storing and manipulating verbal and auditory information. It consists of two subcomponents: the phonological store, which holds information in speech-based form, and the articulatory control process, which allows for rehearsal.

- **The Visuospatial Sketchpad:** Handles visual and spatial information, enabling the manipulation and temporary storage of images and spatial relationships. This component is crucial for tasks such as navigation and understanding graphic patterns.

- **The Episodic Buffer:** Introduced later to the model, the episodic buffer integrates information from the phonological loop, visuospatial sketchpad, and long-term memory into a coherent episode. Its multidimensional code allows it to hold and combine information from different sources.

Functioning of Working Memory

Working memory plays a pivotal role in daily cognitive functions:

- **Language Comprehension:** It holds and manipulates the information needed to understand sentences and discourse.

- **Learning:** It temporarily stores new information for integration into long-term memory.

- **Reasoning and Decision Making:** It holds relevant information in an accessible state for evaluating options and consequences.

- **Attentional Control:** The central executive directs focus and allocates cognitive resources according to task demands.

Neural Basis of Working Memory

Neuroimaging studies have identified several brain regions associated with working memory functions:

- **Prefrontal Cortex:** Critical for the central executive functions, involved in the planning, initiating, and regulating cognitive tasks.

- **Parietal Lobes:** Involved in the visuospatial sketchpad, playing a role in spatial attention and manipulation.

- **Temporal Lobes:** Associated with the phonological loop, particularly in storing and manipulating verbal information.

Limitations and Capacity

Working memory has limited capacity, which varies among individuals and can be affected by age, cognitive development, and neurological conditions. Strategies such as chunking (grouping information into larger units) and rehearsal can enhance working memory efficiency.

Impact on Learning and Cognitive Development

Working memory capacity strongly predicts academic achievement, particularly in reading comprehension and mathematics. Deficits in working memory are linked to difficulties in learning and are characteristic of several cognitive disorders, including ADHD and dyslexia.

In summary, working memory is a foundational human cognition component underpinning our ability to process, store, and manipulate information in real-time. Its effective functioning is essential for a wide range of cognitive activities, from basic comprehension to complex problem-solving, highlighting its importance in cognitive psychology and neuroscience.

6.3 Decision-Making and Problem-Solving

Decision-making and problem-solving are integral cognitive processes that enable individuals to choose between alternatives and solve complex issues. These processes are underpinned by a combination of cognitive functions, including attention, working memory, and executive functions, and are influenced by both rational analysis and emotional responses.

Decision Making

Decision-making involves choosing between two or more alternatives, often under conditions of uncertainty. It encompasses several models and theories:

- **Rational Decision Making:** Assumes that individuals make decisions by systematically evaluating all alternatives and their outcomes to select the best option. This model emphasizes logical and structured analysis.

- **Heuristics and Biases:** Heuristics are mental shortcuts that simplify decision-making but can lead to systematic errors or biases. Common heuristics include the availability heuristic (basing decisions on readily available information) and the representativeness heuristic (judging probabilities based on similarities to existing prototypes).

- **Dual-Process Theories:** Suggest that decision-making involves two distinct systems: an intuitive, fast, and automatic system (System 1) and a deliberate, slow, and controlled system (System 2). These systems can sometimes compete, leading to conflicts in decision-making.

Problem Solving

Problem-solving is the process of finding solutions to difficult or complex issues. It involves several stages:

- **Problem Identification:** Recognizing and defining the problem.

- **Strategy Formulation:** Developing strategies or approaches to solve the problem.

- **Organizing Information:** Gathering and structuring relevant information using working memory and attention.

- **Allocation of Resources:** Deciding how much time and effort to allocate to different strategies.

- **Implementation:** Applying strategies to solve the problem.

- **Evaluation:** Assessing the solution's effectiveness and revising strategies as necessary.

Cognitive Strategies in Problem Solving

Several strategies are employed in problem-solving, including:

- **Algorithm:** A step-by-step procedure that guarantees a solution but may be time-consuming.

- **Heuristic:** A general problem-solving framework that is quicker but does not guarantee a correct solution.

- **Insight:** A sudden realization of a problem's solution, often called an "aha" moment.

- **Trial and Error:** Trying different solutions until one works is valuable when the number of potential solutions is limited.

Factors Influencing Decision Making and Problem Solving

- **Cognitive Biases:** Preconceived notions and biases can influence decision-making and problem-solving, leading to suboptimal outcomes.

- **Emotional Factors:** Emotions play a significant role in decision-making, influencing preferences and risk perception.

- **Social Influences:** Decisions and problem-solving strategies can be affected by social context, norms, and pressures.

- **Individual Differences:** Variability in cognitive abilities, such as working memory capacity and fluid intelligence, can impact an individual's effectiveness in decision-making and problem-solving.

Neurocognitive Aspects

Neuroimaging studies have identified several brain regions involved in decision-making and problem-solving, including the prefrontal cortex (executive functions), the amygdala (emotional responses), and the parietal cortex (information processing).

Understanding the cognitive processes underlying decision-making and problem-solving provides insights into human behavior and cognition and has practical implications for education, business, and therapy. By recognizing the factors that influence these processes, individuals can develop strategies to improve their decision-making and problem-solving abilities, leading to more effective outcomes in various aspects of life.

6.4 Exercise: 10 MCQs with Answers at the End

Test your understanding of decision-making, problem-solving, and their cognitive underpinnings with the following multiple-choice questions. Answers are provided at the end for self-assessment.

1. What type of decision-making model assumes individuals evaluate all alternatives to select the best one?

   - A) Rational decision making

   - B) Heuristics and biases

   - C) Dual-process theories

   - D) Emotional decision-making

2. Which heuristic is based on the ease with which instances come to mind?

   - A) Availability heuristic

   - B) Representativeness heuristic

   - C) Anchoring heuristic

   - D) Adjustment heuristic

3. System 1 decision-making is characterized as:

- A) Slow and controlled

- B) Fast and automatic

- C) Sequential and logical

- D) Reflective and analytical

4. The process of finding solutions to difficult or complex issues is known as:

- A) Decision making

- B) Problem-solving

- C) Cognitive biasing

- D) Heuristic processing

5. What is the sudden realization of a problem's solution often referred to as?

- A) Algorithm

- B) Heuristic

- C) Insight

- D) Trial and Error

6. Which of the following is NOT a stage in problem-solving?

- A) Problem identification

- B) Strategy formulation

- C) Emotional regulation

- D) Implementation

7. Emotional influences in decision-making primarily affect:

  - A) Preferences and risk perception

  - B) Algorithmic processing

  - C) Logical reasoning

  - D) Sequential analysis

8. What role does the prefrontal cortex play in decision-making and problem-solving?

  - A) Emotional responses

  - B) Executive functions

  - C) Sensory processing

  - D) Motor coordination

9. Trial and error is a problem-solving strategy that is most useful when:

  - A) There are a limited number of solutions

  - B) A precise and guaranteed solution is needed

  - C) The problem is well-defined and structured

  - D) There is ample time for problem-solving

10. Which cognitive process is crucial for organizing and structuring relevant information during problem-solving?

   - A) Working memory

   - B) Long-term memory

   - C) Sensory memory

   - D) Implicit memory

Answers:

1. A) Rational decision making

2. A) Availability heuristic

3. B) Fast and automatic

4. B) Problem solving

5. C) Insight

6. C) Emotional regulation

7. A) Preferences and risk perception

8. B) Executive functions

9. A) There are a limited number of solutions

10. A) Working memory

These questions assess your knowledge of the cognitive processes involved in decision-making and problem-solving, including the models, heuristics, and brain regions associated with these complex activities. Reviewing your answers will help you gauge your understanding of these concepts and identify areas for further exploration or study.

Chapter 7: Emotions and the Brain

7.1 The Neuroscience of Emotions

Emotions are complex psychological states that involve a coordinated set of responses by the brain and body to significant internal thoughts or external stimuli. These responses can include physiological arousal, expressive behaviors, and conscious experience. Understanding the neuroscience of emotions involves exploring the brain structures and neural pathways that mediate emotional experiences and expressions.

Key Brain Structures in Emotion

Several brain structures play critical roles in the processing and regulation of emotions:

- **Amygdala:** Central to processing emotions like fear and pleasure. It evaluates the emotional relevance of stimuli and is involved in forming emotional memories. The amygdala plays a crucial role in fear conditioning, helping to associate specific stimuli with fearful or threatening outcomes.

-

Hypothalamus: Regulates physiological responses to emotional stimuli, including the activation of the autonomic nervous and endocrine systems, influencing stress responses, sexual arousal, and aggression.

- **Hippocampus:** Involved in forming, organizing, and storing emotionally charged memories. It works closely with the amygdala to link specific contexts to emotional experiences.

- **Prefrontal Cortex (PFC):** Plays a crucial role in regulating emotional responses and decision-making processes involving dynamic information. The PFC is involved in the inhibition of inappropriate emotional reactions and the modulation of passionate intensity. It also contributes to empathy, guilt, and moral judgment.

- **Anterior Cingulate Cortex (ACC):** Involved in the emotional aspect of pain perception, empathy, and decision-making. The ACC helps to assess the emotional significance of events and errors, and it plays a role in emotional regulation and detecting conflicts.

- **Insula:** Important for the subjective experience of emotions, such as disgust, and the perception of bodily states associated with emotions, contributing to the gut feeling.

Neural Pathways for Emotion

Emotions are the result of complex interactions among various brain regions. Two primary pathways are involved in the processing of emotional stimuli:

- **The Low Road:** A fast, automatic pathway that processes emotional stimuli subconsciously, allowing for quick responses to potentially threatening situations. This pathway involves direct connections from the thalamus to the amygdala.

- **The High Road:** A slower, more deliberate pathway that involves conscious processing of emotional stimuli. It includes the sensory, hippocampus, and prefrontal cortex, allowing for a more nuanced evaluation and response to emotional stimuli.

The Role of Neurotransmitters and Hormones

Various neurotransmitters and hormones also influence emotional responses:

- **Dopamine:** Associated with pleasure and reward.

- **Serotonin:** Linked to mood regulation, with low levels associated with depression.

- **Norepinephrine:** Influences arousal and alertness.

- **Cortisol:** A stress hormone released in response to perceived threats, affecting memory, immune function, and metabolism.

Emotions and Mental Health

Dysregulation of emotional processing can lead to various mental health disorders, such as anxiety disorders, depression, and PTSD. Understanding the neuroscience of emotions is crucial for developing effective treatments for these conditions, including psychotherapy, medication, and neuromodulation techniques.

In summary, the neuroscience of emotions encompasses the study of brain structures, neural pathways, neurotransmitters, and hormones that mediate emotions' complex experiences. This field advances our understanding of the human emotional experience and informs clinical practices for emotional and psychological well-being.

7.2 Emotion Regulation

Emotion regulation refers to the processes by which individuals influence which emotions they have, when they have them, and how they experience and express these emotions. It is crucial to mental health and well-being, impacting interpersonal relationships, decision-making, and overall psychological resilience. Emotion regulation involves both automatic and controlled processes that can modulate emotional responses at various stages of the emotion generation process.

Strategies for Emotion Regulation

Several strategies have been identified for regulating emotions, each with different implications for psychological well-being:

- **Cognitive Reappraisal:** Involves changing the way one thinks about a potentially emotion-eliciting situation to alter its emotional impact. It is considered an adaptive strategy associated with better psychological health.

- **Suppression:** Entails inhibiting the outward signs of emotion, which can reduce the expression of emotion but does not decrease the emotional experience. Suppression is generally viewed as less adaptive, as it can increase stress and reduce social connectedness.

- **Distraction:** Diverting attention away from the emotional stimulus to neutral or pleasant stimuli can effectively reduce the intensity of emotional responses, especially in the short term.

- **Acceptance:** Involves acknowledging and accepting emotions as they are, without trying to change or judge them. Acceptance is a cornerstone of mindfulness and is associated with greater emotional and psychological well-being.

Neural Bases of Emotion Regulation

Neuroscience research has begun to elucidate the brain mechanisms underlying emotion regulation, highlighting the involvement of several key regions:

- **Prefrontal Cortex (PFC):** The PFC, especially the ventrolateral and dorsolateral regions, plays a critical role in the cognitive control of emotion, including strategies like reappraisal and suppression. It is involved in planning, decision-making, and moderating social behavior.

- **Anterior Cingulate Cortex (ACC):** The ACC monitors emotional responses and detects conflicts between emotional impulses and regulatory goals.

- **Amygdala:** Although primarily involved in emotion generation, the amygdala also interacts with prefrontal regions to regulate emotions, often modulated by cognitive reappraisal strategies.

Impact of Emotion Regulation on Mental Health

Effective emotion regulation strategies can buffer against mental health disorders and enhance psychological resilience. Difficulty in regulating emotions is a common feature across various psychiatric conditions, including depression, anxiety disorders, and borderline personality disorder. Interventions aimed at improving emotion regulation skills, such as cognitive-behavioral therapy (CBT) and dialectical behavior therapy (DBT), are effective in treating these conditions.

Development of Emotion Regulation

The ability to regulate emotions develops throughout childhood and adolescence, influenced by genetic factors, socialization processes, and environmental experiences. Parenting styles, social interactions, and cultural norms significantly shape emotion regulation strategies and competencies.

In summary, emotion regulation is a complex process involving the modulation of emotional experiences and expressions through various cognitive and behavioral strategies. Understanding the mechanisms of emotion regulation and the role of specific brain regions in this process is crucial for psychological research and clinical practice, offering insights into managing emotional responses and treating emotional disorders.

7.3 The Role of Emotions in Decision-Making

Emotions play a pivotal role in decision-making, influencing our choices and how we make them. Traditionally, emotions were often viewed as impediments to rational decision-making. However, contemporary research in psychology and neuroscience has revealed that emotions are integral to the decision-making process, providing critical information about our preferences, values, and potential outcomes of our choices.

The Dual-Process Model of Decision Making

The dual-process model, which distinguishes between System 1 (intuitive and emotional) and System 2 (analytical and deliberate) processes, underscores the interplay between emotion and cognition in decision-making. Emotions are primarily associated with System 1, guiding decisions through gut feelings or intuitive judgments, while System 2 involves more rational and calculated evaluation.

How Emotions Influence Decision-Making

- **Emotional Markers:** Antonio Damasio's somatic marker hypothesis suggests that emotional reactions to specific experiences are stored as somatic markers associated with those experiences. These markers then influence future decision-making by signaling potential outcomes and guiding individuals towards advantageous choices and away from detrimental ones.

- **Risk Assessment:** Emotions significantly affect how people perceive and respond to risk. Fear can lead to risk-averse behaviors, while happiness or excitement might make individuals more open to taking risks.

- **Motivation and Goals:** Desires and aversions, shaped by emotional experiences, influence goal-directed behavior. Emotions can motivate individuals to pursue specific goals and avoid others, impacting decision-making strategies and outcomes.

- **Social and Moral Decision Making:** Emotions are crucial in social interactions and moral judgments. Empathy, guilt, and anger, for example, can profoundly influence decisions in social contexts, affecting behaviors such as cooperation, altruism, and punishment.

Impact of Emotional Regulation on Decision-Making

The ability to regulate emotions is essential for adaptive decision-making. Effective emotion regulation can enhance decision-making by allowing for a balanced consideration of emotional and rational perspectives. Conversely, difficulties in emotion regulation can lead to impulsive, short-sighted, or maladaptive decisions.

Neuroscience Perspective

Neuroimaging studies have illuminated the neural correlates of the interaction between emotion and decision-making. Key regions involved include:

- **The Prefrontal Cortex (PFC):** Involved in emotional regulation and rational decision-making, the PFC helps integrate dynamic inputs with cognitive processes.

- **The Amygdala:** Plays a central role in emotional processing and has been linked to decision-making under uncertainty and assessing rewards and punishments.

- **The Insula:** Associated with the subjective experience of emotions, the insula is mainly involved in risk, loss aversion, and disgust decisions.

Emotions in Economic Decision Making

The field of behavioral economics integrates psychological insights into economic theory, highlighting how emotions can lead to deviations from what traditional economic models would predict as 'rational' behavior. Emotions can lead to biases such as overvaluing immediate rewards over future gains (present bias) or the tendency to stick with the status quo (status quo bias).

In summary, emotions are integral to decision-making, providing crucial information that guides our choices, influences our perception of risk, and motivates our goals and behaviors. Understanding the role of emotions in decision-making is essential for fields ranging from psychology and neuroscience to economics and business, highlighting the complex interplay between emotion and cognition in shaping human behavior.

7.4 Exercise: 10 MCQs with Answers at the End

Test your knowledge of the role of emotions in the brain, emotion regulation, and their impact on decision-making with these multiple-choice questions. Answers are provided at the end for self-assessment.

1. Which brain structure is primarily associated with the processing of fear and pleasure?

   - A) Hippocampus

   - B) Amygdala

   - C) Prefrontal Cortex

   - D) Anterior Cingulate Cortex

2. The somatic marker hypothesis, which suggests that emotional reactions guide decision-making, was proposed by:

- A) Daniel Kahneman

- B) Antonio Damasio

- C) B.F. Skinner

- D) Carl Rogers

3. Which of the following is NOT a strategy for emotion regulation?

- A) Cognitive reappraisal

- B) Suppression

- C) Distraction

- D) Procrastination

4. Emotions can influence decision-making by:

- A) Decreasing risk perception

- B) Eliminating cognitive biases

- C) Signaling potential outcomes through somatic markers

- D) Always leading to rational choices

5. The ability to maintain attention on a task over an extended period is known as:

- A) Selective attention

- B) Sustained attention

- C) Divided attention

- D) Executive attention

6. Which brain area is involved in the cognitive control of emotions and decision-making processes?

- A) Amygdala

- B) Hippocampus

- C) Prefrontal Cortex

- D) Insula

7. What role does the anterior cingulate cortex (ACC) play in emotion?

- A) It processes visual and emotional stimuli.

- B) It is involved in emotional regulation and detecting conflicts.

- C) It stores emotional memories.

- D) It directly processes fear responses.

8. Distraction as an emotion regulation strategy involves:

   - A) Changing the way one thinks about an emotion-eliciting situation

   - B) Inhibiting outward signs of emotion

   - C) Shifting attention away from the emotional stimulus

   - D) Accepting emotions as they are

9. System 1 decision making is characterized by:

   - A) Being slow and deliberate

   - B) Relying on logical analysis

   - C) Being fast and based on emotional responses

   - D) The absence of biases

10. Effective emotion regulation is associated with:

   - A) Increased psychological stress

   - B) Decreased social connectivity

   - C) Better psychological health

   - D) Impaired decision-making skills

Answers:

1. B) Amygdala

2. B) Antonio Damasio

3. D) Procrastination

4. C) Signaling potential outcomes through somatic markers

5. B) Sustained attention

6. C) Prefrontal Cortex

7. B) It is involved in emotional regulation and detecting conflicts.

8. C) Shifting attention away from the emotional stimulus

9. C) Being fast and based on emotional responses

10. C) Better psychological health

These questions are designed to test your understanding of the neuroscience of emotions, how emotions are regulated, and their significant influence on decision-making processes. Reviewing your answers will help you gauge your grasp of these complex topics and identify areas for further exploration.

Chapter 8: Social Cognition

8.1 Theory of Mind

Theory of Mind (ToM) is a fundamental aspect of social cognition, referring to the ability to attribute mental states—beliefs, intents, desires, emotions, knowledge—to oneself and others. This capacity enables individuals to understand that others have thoughts, feelings, and perspectives that are different from their own, facilitating complex social interactions and empathetic engagement.

Development of Theory of Mind

The development of ToM is a critical milestone in child development, typically emerging around the age of 4 or 5 years. Early signs of ToM can be observed in infants, suggesting a rudimentary understanding of others' actions and intentions. Vital developmental milestones include:

- **Understanding False Beliefs:** The classic test of ToM is the false belief task, where children must predict a character's action based on the character's belief, which differs from the child's knowledge. Success in this task indicates an understanding that others can hold incorrect assumptions about the world.

- **Perspective Taking:** The ability to view situations from another person's perspective, understanding that different people may see things differently based on their beliefs and experiences.

- **Understanding Emotions:** Recognizing that others have their emotional responses that may differ from one's own and that beliefs and desires can influence these responses.

Components of Theory of Mind

ToM encompasses several components, including:

- **Cognitive ToM:** The ability to understand others' beliefs, thoughts, and intentions.

- **Affective ToM:** The capacity to infer and understand others' emotions and feelings.

- **Social Perception:** The skill to interpret social cues such as facial expressions, tone of voice, and body language, which are critical for inferring mental states.

Neural Bases of Theory of Mind

Neuroimaging studies have identified several brain regions involved in ToM, including:

- **The Medial Prefrontal Cortex (mPFC):** Associated with thinking about oneself and others' mental states.

- **The Temporo-Parietal Junction (TPJ):** Involved in understanding others' perspectives and intentions.

- **The Superior Temporal Sulcus (STS):** Plays a role in interpreting social cues and actions.

- **The Amygdala:** Important for processing emotional aspects of ToM.

Theory of Mind and Social Functioning

ToM is crucial for effective social functioning, allowing individuals to engage in social reasoning, predict others' behavior, and navigate the social world. Deficits in ToM are associated with social-communication difficulties, as seen in autism spectrum disorder (ASD) and schizophrenia, where individuals may struggle to infer others' mental states or understand social cues.

Theory of Mind in Adults

While ToM is most commonly studied in the context of child development, it plays a significant role throughout adulthood, influencing social interactions, empathy, moral reasoning, and conflict resolution.

In summary, the Theory of Mind is a cornerstone of social cognition, enabling individuals to understand and predict the mental states of others. Its development is a complex process influenced by biological, cognitive, and social factors, and it underpins many aspects of social interaction and communication.

8.2 Empathy and Moral Reasoning

Empathy

Empathy is the ability to understand and share the feelings of another person. It's a foundational component of social cognition that facilitates interpersonal connections, compassion, and altruistic behavior. Empathy can be divided into two main types:

- **Cognitive Empathy:** Also known as perspective-taking, cognitive empathy refers to the ability to understand another person's mental state or viewpoint without necessarily sharing their emotions. It involves recognizing and reasoning about others' thoughts, beliefs, and intentions.

- **Affective Empathy:** This type of empathy involves sharing another person's emotional experience. It's the capacity to feel what another person is feeling or to respond to the affective state of another individual emotionally.

Empathy is not just a passive process; it influences how we interact with others, informing our responses and behaviors in social contexts.

Neural Bases of Empathy

Empathy engages multiple brain regions and networks, including:

- **The Mirror Neuron System:** Involved in understanding the actions and intentions of others and thought to be a mechanism by which we simulate others' experiences.

- **The Insula:** Plays a vital role in the subjective experience of emotions and is involved in affective empathy, particularly in feeling the feelings of others.

- **The Anterior Cingulate Cortex (ACC)** Associated with the affective component of empathy and the emotional response to others' pain or distress.

- **The Medial Prefrontal Cortex (mPFC):** Involved in cognitive empathy and perspective-taking, facilitating understanding of others' mental states.

Moral Reasoning

Moral reasoning is how individuals decide right and wrong, good and bad. It involves the application of moral principles and values to specific situations, guiding ethical behavior and judgments.

- **Kohlberg's Stages of Moral Development:** Lawrence Kohlberg proposed a theory of moral development that outlines three levels and six stages through which individuals progress as they mature. These stages move from focusing on obedience and punishment through a social-order maintaining orientation to principled moral reasoning based on abstract ethical principles.

- **The Role of Emotions in Moral Reasoning:** Emotions play a significant role in moral reasoning, influencing judgments and decisions. For example, feelings of empathy, guilt, or anger can impact how we perceive moral dilemmas and guide our ethical behavior.

Interplay Between Empathy and Moral Reasoning

Empathy and moral reasoning are closely linked, with empathy often providing the emotional foundation for moral concern and ethical behavior. Empathy can motivate prosocial behavior and moral action by making the welfare of others salient and personally meaningful.

- **Empathy-Induced Altruism:** The emotional response elicited by empathy can lead to altruistic behavior, where actions are taken to benefit another person, even at a cost to oneself.

- **Moral Dilemmas:** In complex moral dilemmas, empathy can influence moral reasoning by highlighting the emotional consequences of actions, thereby affecting ethical decisions.

In summary, empathy and moral reasoning are integral components of social cognition, profoundly intertwined and critical for understanding and navigating the social world. They underpin our ability to connect with others, make ethical decisions, and engage in prosocial behavior. The study of these processes not only provides insights into human social behavior and has implications for education, psychology, and ethics.

8.3 Social Influence on Behavior

Social influence encompasses how individuals change their behavior to meet the demands of a social environment. It plays a critical role in human behavior, shaping everything from the mundane to the significant, influencing our choices, beliefs, and attitudes. Understanding social influence involves examining the various mechanisms through which people are affected by the presence, actions, or expectations of others.

Types of Social Influence

- **Conformity:** The change in behavior or belief due to natural or imagined group pressure. Solomon Asch's experiments on conformity demonstrated how individuals often conform to group norms even when they privately disagree, highlighting the powerful effect of the need for social acceptance.

- **Compliance:** changing one's behavior in response to a direct request. Techniques such as the "foot-in-the-door" (making a small request followed by a larger one) and the "door-in-the-face" (making an unreasonably large request followed by a smaller one) effectively illustrate how compliance can be achieved.

- **Obedience:** A form of social influence where an individual follows an authority figure's direct order or command. Stanley Milgram's obedience experiments showcased the extent to which individuals are willing to obey authority figures, even when asked to perform actions conflicting with their conscience.

- **Persuasion:** The process of changing attitudes, beliefs, or behaviors through argument, reasoning, or appeal. Factors that affect persuasion include the message's source, the message itself, and the audience's characteristics.

Mechanisms of Social Influence

Social influence operates through several mechanisms:

- **Normative Social Influence:** The influence to conform to the positive expectations of others, driven by the desire to be liked and accepted by the group.

- **Informational Social Influence:** Stemming from the desire to be correct in situations where the proper action or belief is uncertain, leading individuals to conform to group behavior.

The Role of Social Context

The impact of social influence can vary significantly depending on the context, including:

- **Group Size and Unanimity:** Larger groups and unanimous opinions tend to increase conformity, though there are diminishing returns as group size increases beyond a certain point.

- **Cultural Factors:** Collectivist cultures, which emphasize group harmony and consensus, may exhibit higher conformity and obedience than individualistic cultures.

- **Social Roles and Identities:** Individuals' social roles and identification with specific groups can significantly influence their behavior and susceptibility to social influence.

Social Influence in Everyday Life

Social influence is pervasive, affecting various aspects of daily life, such as consumer behavior, political opinions, and social norms. Understanding these influences can help individuals recognize the factors shaping their behavior and make more informed choices.

In summary, social influence is a fundamental aspect of social cognition, affecting how individuals think, feel, and behave within a social context. By examining conformity, compliance, obedience, and persuasion, we gain insights into human behavior's complex dynamics and the social environment's powerful impact.

8.4 Exercise: 10 MCQs with Answers at the End

Test your knowledge of social cognition, including theory of mind, empathy, moral reasoning, and social influence on behavior, with these multiple-choice questions. Answers are provided at the end for self-assessment.

1. Theory of Mind is best described as:

   - A) The cognitive ability to reason about physics.

   - B) The understanding that other people have their thoughts, feelings, and perspectives.

   - C) The skill of memorizing social information.

   - D) The ability to solve complex mathematical problems.

2. Which type of empathy involves understanding another person's emotional state without necessarily feeling it yourself?

   - A) Affective empathy

   - B) Cognitive empathy

   - C) Sympathetic empathy

   - D) Compassionate empathy

3. Lawrence Kohlberg is known for his theory of:

   - A) Cognitive development.

   - B) Moral development.

   - C) Social influence.

   - D) Emotional intelligence.

4. Conformity is most closely related to:

   - A) Changing one's behavior due to a direct order from an authority.

   - B) Changing one's behavior in response to a request.

   - C) Changing one's behavior to align with group norms.

   - D) Changing one's beliefs after being persuaded.

5. The "foot-in-the-door" technique is a strategy used in:

   - A) Obedience

   - B) Compliance

   - C) Conformity

   - D) Persuasion

6. The neural basis of empathy involves all the following brain regions EXCEPT:

   - A) The amygdala

   - B) The hippocampus

   - C) The insula

   - D) The anterior cingulate cortex

7. Social influence that stems from the desire to be correct in ambiguous situations is called:

- A) Normative social influence

- B) Informational social influence

- C) Conformity pressure

- D) Authoritative demand

8. Which experiment is famously associated with studying obedience to authority?

- A) The Stanford prison experiment

- B) The Asch conformity experiments

- C) The Milgram experiment

- D) The Marshmallow test

9. Persuasion is the process of:

- A) Forcing someone to accept your point of view.

- B) Changing attitudes or behaviors through reasoning or appeal.

- C) Using authority to change beliefs.

- D) Following social norms without questioning.

10. The ability to feel what another person is feeling is known as:

   - A) Cognitive empathy

   - B) Affective empathy

   - C) Compassionate empathy

   - D) Emotional intelligence

Answers:

1. B) The understanding that other people have their thoughts, feelings, and perspectives.

2. B) Cognitive empathy

3. B) Moral development.

4. C) Changing one's behavior to align with group norms.

5. B) Compliance

6. B) The hippocampus

7. B) Informational social influence

8. C) The Milgram experiment

9. B) Changing attitudes or behaviors through reasoning or appeal.

10. B) Affective empathy

These questions are designed to test your understanding of various concepts within social cognition, offering insight into how we perceive and interact with the social world around us. Reviewing your answers will help you assess your grasp of these topics and identify areas for further exploration.

Chapter 9: Neurodevelopment and Aging

9.1 Brain Development from Infancy to Adulthood

Brain development is a complex process that begins before birth and continues into adulthood. It involves changes in the brain's size, structure, and function, influenced by a combination of genetic factors and environmental inputs. Understanding the trajectory of brain development from infancy to adulthood provides insights into the neural underpinnings of cognitive, emotional, and social growth.

Prenatal Development

- Brain development starts just a few weeks after conception, with the formation of the neural tube, which eventually becomes the central nervous system (CNS).

- By the end of the first trimester, the brain's basic structure is established, and neurons begin to form at an extraordinary rate.

Infancy and Early Childhood

- The first few years of life are characterized by rapid brain growth, known as the brain's "critical period." The brain is highly plastic during this time, making it susceptible to environmental stimuli. This plasticity allows for rapid motor skills, language, and social behavior development.

- Synaptogenesis, the formation of synapses between neurons, occurs rapidly, peaking around 2-3 years of age. This is followed by synaptic pruning, eliminating unused connections, and making the brain's network more efficient.

Adolescence

- Adolescence marks another significant period of brain development, with notable changes in the structure and activity of the brain, particularly in the prefrontal cortex and limbic system. These changes are associated with improvements in executive functions, such as planning, decision-making, impulse control, and heightened emotional and social sensitivity.

- Myelination, the process of coating the axons of neurons with a fatty substance called myelin, continues during adolescence, enhancing the speed and efficiency of neural communication.

Adulthood

- Brain development in adulthood involves fine-tuning neural circuits and continued plasticity in response to learning and experience.

- While the creation of new neurons (neurogenesis) is limited in most parts of the adult brain, it continues in specific areas, such as the hippocampus, which is involved in learning and memory.

Aging

- As the brain ages, it undergoes structural and functional changes, including brain volume and weight reductions, particularly in the prefrontal cortex and hippocampus.

- Age-related changes also include decreased synaptic density and neurotransmitter system alterations, which can impact cognitive functions. However, cognitive decline is not inevitable, and many individuals maintain high levels of cognitive function well into old age through cognitive reserve. This concept refers to the brain's resilience to neuropathological damage.

Influences on Brain Development

- Genetic factors provide the blueprint for brain development, while environmental factors, such as nutrition, social interactions, and learning experiences, shape how this blueprint is expressed.

- Early life experiences, including exposure to stress or enriched environments, can have long-lasting effects on brain structure and function.

In summary, brain development from infancy to adulthood is a dynamic and prolonged process that lays the foundation for a wide range of cognitive, emotional, and social capabilities. Understanding these developmental trajectories sheds light on the nature of human growth and aging and emphasizes the importance of supportive environments throughout the lifespan for optimal brain health and functioning.

9.2 Cognitive Changes in Aging

As individuals age, they often experience changes in cognitive functions. Cognitive aging is a complex process influenced by various factors, including genetics, lifestyle, and overall brain health. While aging can be associated with cognitive decline in specific domains, it's also characterized by stability or improvement in others. Understanding the nuances of mental changes in aging is essential for promoting healthy cognitive aging.

Domains of Cognitive Change

- **Memory:** Age-related declines are most pronounced in episodic memory, the ability to recall specific events from the past. Older adults may also experience changes in working memory and memory consolidation. However, semantic memory, or knowledge of facts and concepts, tends to remain stable or improve with age.

- **Attention:** While essential attentional capacities are relatively well-preserved, older adults may show declines in divided attention tasks and situations requiring rapid attention shifting.

- **Processing Speed:** One of the most noticeable changes is a reduction in processing speed, the pace at which individuals can understand and respond to information. This slowing can affect cognitive tasks, from simple reaction time to more complex problem-solving activities.

- **Executive Functions:** These include planning, decision-making, error correction, and inhibitory control. While some aspects of executive functioning may decline, others, such as emotional regulation and experience-based problem-solving, often remain stable or improve.

- **Language:** Vocabulary and verbal abilities are areas of strength for many older adults, with improvements or stability well into later life. However, older individuals may experience difficulties with language production, such as finding the right words during conversation.

Factors Influencing Cognitive Aging

- **Biological Factors:** Brain structure and function changes, including brain atrophy, reduced synaptic density, and alterations in neurotransmitter systems, can contribute to cognitive aging.

- **Health Conditions:** Medical conditions such as cardiovascular disease, diabetes, and hypertension, and lifestyle factors like physical activity, diet, and social engagement significantly impact cognitive aging.

- **Cognitive Reserve:** This concept refers to the brain's resilience to neuropathological damage. Individuals with higher cognitive reserve, often due to education, occupational complexity, and engagement in cognitively stimulating activities, may experience slower cognitive decline.

Cognitive Aging and Neurodegenerative Diseases

It's important to differentiate between normal cognitive aging and cognitive changes due to neurodegenerative diseases like Alzheimer's disease or other forms of dementia. While normal aging involves selective changes in specific cognitive domains, neurodegenerative diseases are characterized by more widespread and severe cognitive impairments.

Promoting Healthy Cognitive Aging

Strategies to promote healthy cognitive aging focus on maintaining overall physical health, engaging in regular physical and mental activities, fostering social connections, and managing chronic health conditions. Lifelong learning and engaging in new and challenging activities can also support mental health in later life.

In summary, cognitive changes in aging encompass a broad spectrum of experiences, from declines in certain areas to stability or improvements in others. Understanding these changes is critical to supporting healthy aging, highlighting the importance of a holistic approach that includes physical health, mental stimulation, and social well-being.

9.3 Neuroplasticity across the Lifespan

Neuroplasticity, the brain's ability to reorganize itself by forming new neural connections throughout life, is fundamental to learning, memory, and recovery from brain injuries. Contrary to the once-prevailing belief that the brain's plasticity diminishes with age, current research indicates that neuroplasticity continues across the lifespan, albeit with variations in efficiency and capacity at different stages.

Neuroplasticity in Infancy and Childhood

The brain exhibits a high degree of plasticity during infancy and early childhood. This period is characterized by rapid growth in brain size and complexity, driven by processes such as synaptogenesis (formation of synaptic connections), myelination (formation of myelin sheaths around axons to speed up neural communication), and synaptic pruning (elimination of unused synapses to increase the efficiency of neuronal transmissions).

- **Critical Periods:** There are windows of opportunity, known as critical periods, during which the developing brain is particularly receptive to specific sensory, motor, or cognitive inputs. For instance, language acquisition is most efficient during early childhood.

Neuroplasticity in Adolescence

Adolescence is another crucial period for brain development, marked by continued synaptic pruning and strengthening of connections that are frequently used. These changes contribute to improvements in abstract thinking, decision-making, and self-regulation.

- The prefrontal cortex, responsible for executive functions, undergoes significant reorganization during adolescence, affecting emotional regulation and risk-taking behaviors.

Neuroplasticity in Adulthood

While the rate of neuroplastic changes slows in adulthood, plasticity remains integral to learning and memory. Adult neuroplasticity is often more targeted and specific, requiring more effort and repetition to establish new neural pathways.

- **Lifelong Learning:** Engaging in new learning activities and skills can promote neuroplasticity, contributing to cognitive resilience.

- **Recovery from Injury:** Neuroplasticity plays a crucial role in recovery from brain injuries, with the brain's ability to rewire itself and compensate for damaged areas.

Neuroplasticity and Aging

In older adults, neuroplasticity plays a vital role in maintaining cognitive function and adapting to age-related changes in the brain.

- **Cognitive Reserve:** A higher cognitive reserve, built through a lifetime of education and engaging in mentally stimulating activities, can mitigate the impact of age-related brain changes and reduce the risk of cognitive decline.

- **Physical Exercise:** Regular physical activity has been shown to promote neuroplasticity in older adults, including the growth of new neurons (neurogenesis) in the hippocampus, a region crucial for memory and learning.

Challenges to Neuroplasticity with Age

- While neuroplasticity persists throughout life, the aging brain may face challenges such as reduced synaptic plasticity, slower rates of neurogenesis, and increased susceptibility to neurodegenerative diseases, which can impact the effectiveness of new learning and recovery processes.

In summary, neuroplasticity across the lifespan underscores the brain's remarkable capacity to adapt and reorganize in response to new experiences, learning, and environmental changes. From the rapid developmental changes in early life to the more nuanced adaptations in adulthood and old age, neuroplasticity remains a cornerstone of brain function, highlighting the importance of continued cognitive engagement and physical activity to support brain health and cognitive function at all ages.

9.4 Exercise: 10 MCQs with Answers at the End

These multiple-choice questions test your understanding of neurodevelopment, aging, and neuroplasticity across the lifespan. Answers are provided at the end for self-assessment.

1. Which process is characterized by eliminating unused synapses to increase the efficiency of neuronal transmissions?

   - A) Myelination

   - B) Synaptogenesis

   - C) Synaptic pruning

   - D) Neurogenesis

2. During which developmental period is language acquisition most efficient?

   - A) Infancy and early childhood

   - B) Adolescence

   - C) Early adulthood

   - D) Late adulthood

3. The prefrontal cortex, which undergoes significant reorganization during adolescence, is responsible for:

   - A) Sensory processing

   - B) Motor control

   - C) Executive functions

   - D) Visual perception

4. Lifelong learning and engaging in new activities in adulthood promote:

   - A) Synaptic pruning

   - B) Myelination

   - C) Neuroplasticity

   - D) Neurodegeneration

5. What role does physical exercise play in older adults' neuroplasticity?

   - A) It reduces the rate of synaptic pruning.

 - B) It promotes the growth of new neurons in the hippocampus.

   - C) It decreases the efficiency of synaptic transmissions.

   - D) It inhibits the reorganization of neural circuits.

6. Critical periods in brain development are times when:

   - A) The brain is resistant to change.

   - B) Specific types of learning and development are most effective.

   - C) Cognitive decline begins.

   - D) The brain reaches its maximum size.

7. Cognitive reserve can help mitigate the impact of:

   - A) Neurogenesis

   - B) Age-related brain changes

   - C) The critical period of language acquisition

   - D) Synaptogenesis

8. Which factor is NOT directly associated with promoting neuroplasticity in adulthood?

   - A) Regular physical activity

   - B) Engaging in mentally stimulating activities

   - C) Maintaining a high-calorie diet

   - D) Learning new skills

9. Recovery from brain injury in adults showcases the brain's ability to:

   - A) Permanently lose synaptic connections

   - B) Rewire itself and compensate for damaged areas

   - C) Stop the process of myelination

   - D) Increase the rate of neurodegeneration

10. Which of the following best describes neuroplasticity?

   - A) The brain's capacity to degrade with age

   - B) The ability of the brain to reorganize itself by forming new neural connections throughout life

   - C) The process of losing neuronal connections as one age

   - D) The brain's resistance to environmental influences

Answers:

1. C) Synaptic pruning

2. A) Infancy and early childhood

3. C) Executive functions

4. C) Neuroplasticity

5. B) It promotes the growth of new neurons in the hippocampus.

6. B) Specific types of learning and development are most effective.

7. B) Age-related brain changes

8. C) Maintaining a high-calorie diet

9. B) Rewire itself and compensate for damaged areas

10. B) The ability of the brain to reorganize itself by forming new neural connections throughout life

These questions are designed to assess your knowledge of the critical concepts related to brain development, cognitive changes in aging, and the principles of neuroplasticity across the lifespan. Reviewing your answers will help you understand the complexities of neurodevelopment and the brain's adaptability from infancy through old age.

Chapter 10: Neuropsychological Disorders

10.1 Understanding Mental Illness

Mental illnesses, also known as psychiatric disorders, encompass a wide range of conditions that affect mood, thinking, behavior, and perception. These disorders can significantly impact an individual's ability to function in daily life, affecting relationships, work, and overall well-being. Understanding mental illness involves recognizing its complexity, the factors that contribute to its development, and its manifestations.

Classification of Mental Illness

Mental illnesses are classified into several major categories, including but not limited to:

- **Mood Disorders:** Characterized by significant changes or disturbances in mood, examples include major depressive disorder and bipolar disorder.

- **Anxiety Disorders:** Include conditions such as generalized anxiety disorder, panic disorder, and social anxiety disorder, characterized by excessive fear or anxiety.

- **Psychotic Disorders:** Involve distorted thinking and awareness, with schizophrenia being the most notable example, characterized by delusions, hallucinations, and disorganized speech.

- **Personality Disorders:** Patterns of thinking, feeling, and behaving that deviate significantly from cultural expectations, affecting personal and social functioning. Examples include borderline personality disorder and antisocial personality disorder.

- **Eating Disorders:** Involve extreme emotions, attitudes, and behaviors surrounding weight and food issues. Anorexia nervosa and bulimia nervosa are prime examples.

- **Obsessive-Compulsive and Related Disorders:** Characterized by the presence of obsessions (repetitive, intrusive thoughts) and compulsions (repetitive behaviors) aimed at reducing anxiety. Obsessive-compulsive disorder (OCD) falls into this category.

Causes and Risk Factors

The development of mental illness is believed to result from a complex interplay of genetic, biological, environmental, and psychological factors:

- **Genetic Factors:** Many mental illnesses have a hereditary component, suggesting genes play a role in increasing the risk of developing these conditions.

- **Neurobiological Factors:** Imbalances in neurotransmitters and structural or functional abnormalities in specific brain areas can contribute to the manifestation of psychiatric symptoms.

- **Environmental Factors:** Life experiences, including trauma, abuse, and chronic stress, can trigger or exacerbate mental health disorders.

- **Psychological Factors:** Personality traits, coping mechanisms, and early psychological development also influence the risk of developing mental illnesses.

Diagnosis and Treatment

Diagnosing mental illness typically involves a comprehensive assessment that may include physical exams, psychological evaluations, and, in some cases, neuroimaging or other diagnostic tests to rule out other conditions. Treatment approaches vary depending on the disorder and the individual's needs, often involving a combination of:

- **Psychotherapy:** Various forms of therapy, such as cognitive-behavioral therapy (CBT), psychodynamic therapy, and family therapy, can provide individuals with strategies to cope with their condition, understand their thoughts and behaviors, and improve their social functioning.

- **Medication:** Psychiatric medications, including antidepressants, antipsychotics, and anxiolytics, can help manage symptoms by altering brain chemistry.

- **Lifestyle and Supportive Therapies:** Lifestyle changes, peer support, and community services can play critical roles in recovery and ongoing management of mental health conditions.

Understanding mental illness is essential for reducing stigma, promoting empathy, and improving the availability and quality of care for those affected. With advances in research and a growing awareness of the importance of mental health, there is increasing hope for effective treatments and support systems for individuals living with mental illnesses.

10.2 Major Neuropsychological Disorders

Neuropsychological disorders encompass a range of conditions that affect the brain and nervous system, leading to cognitive, emotional, and behavioral impairments. These disorders can arise from various causes, including genetic factors, brain injury, neurological diseases, and environmental influences. Understanding major neuropsychological disorders is crucial for diagnosis, management, and treatment and for developing strategies to support affected individuals and their families.

Alzheimer's Disease (AD)

Alzheimer's disease is a progressive neurodegenerative disorder characterized by the deterioration of memory, thinking, and behavior. It is the most common cause of dementia among older adults. Key features include the accumulation of amyloid-beta plaques and tau protein tangles in the brain, leading to neuronal death and brain atrophy, particularly in the hippocampus and cortex.

Parkinson's Disease (PD)

Parkinson's disease is a chronic and progressive movement disorder resulting from the degeneration of dopamine-producing neurons in the substantia nigra, a region of the midbrain. Symptoms include tremors, rigidity, bradykinesia (slow movement), and postural instability. Cognitive impairments and mood disorders may also develop as the disease progresses.

Stroke

A stroke occurs when the blood supply to part of the brain is interrupted or reduced, preventing brain tissue from receiving oxygen and nutrients. Strokes can lead to a wide range of neuropsychological impairments, depending on the affected brain area, including paralysis, speech and language difficulties, memory and attention deficits, and emotional disturbances.

Traumatic Brain Injury (TBI)

Traumatic brain injury results from a blow or jolt to the head or a penetrating head injury that disrupts normal brain function. TBI can range from mild (concussion) to severe, leading to long-term cognitive, physical, and emotional impairments, such as memory loss, impaired executive functions, mood swings, and personality changes.

Schizophrenia

Schizophrenia is a chronic and severe mental disorder characterized by distortions in thinking, perception, emotions, language, sense of self, and behavior. Symptoms are typically divided into positive symptoms (hallucinations, delusions), negative symptoms (apathy, lack of emotion), and cognitive symptoms (impaired executive function, attention, and working memory).

Autism Spectrum Disorder (ASD)

Autism spectrum disorder is a developmental disorder that affects communication and behavior, with symptoms appearing in the early developmental period. ASD is characterized by difficulties in social interaction, communication challenges, and repetitive behaviors or restricted interests. Cognitive abilities in individuals with ASD can range from severely challenged to above average.

Attention-Deficit/Hyperactivity Disorder (ADHD)

ADHD is a neurodevelopmental disorder characterized by a persistent pattern of inattention and hyperactivity-impulsivity that interferes with functioning or development. It affects children and adults and can lead to academic, occupational, and social difficulties.

Treatment and Management

Treatment of neuropsychological disorders often involves a multidisciplinary approach, including medication, psychotherapy, rehabilitation therapies, and support services. Early diagnosis and intervention are critical for managing symptoms, slowing disease progression, and improving quality of life.

In summary, major neuropsychological disorders encompass a wide range of conditions that can significantly impact cognitive function, emotional well-being, and daily living. Advances in neuroscience and clinical psychology continue to enhance our understanding of these disorders, leading to better diagnostic tools, treatments, and support mechanisms for affected individuals and their families.

10.3 The Impact of Brain Injury

Brain injury, encompassing traumatic brain injury (TBI) and acquired brain injuries (ABI), such as strokes or infections, can have profound and wide-ranging effects on an individual's physical, cognitive, emotional, and social functioning. The impact of brain injury varies significantly based on the severity, location, and nature of the injury, as well as the individual's pre-injury health and cognitive status. Understanding the consequences of brain injury is crucial for providing appropriate care, rehabilitation, and support to affected individuals.

Physical Effects

- **Motor Function:** Brain injuries can lead to paralysis, weakness, poor coordination, and spasticity, affecting mobility and the ability to perform everyday tasks.

- **Sensory Impairments:** Individuals may experience changes in vision, hearing, taste, smell, and touch sensitivity. Visual-perceptual difficulties are expected, including problems with depth perception and spatial orientation.

- **Speech and Language:** Brain injuries can result in aphasia, dysarthria, or other communication disorders, impacting the ability to understand and produce language.

Cognitive Effects

- **Memory:** Short-term and long-term memory can be affected, leading to difficulties in learning new information and recalling past events.

- **Attention and Concentration:** Individuals may have trouble focusing, sustaining, or dividing attention, impacting their ability to complete tasks.

- **Executive Functions:** Impairments in planning, organizing, problem-solving, and decision-making are common, affecting the ability to manage daily activities and responsibilities.

- **Processing Speed:** The speed at which information is processed may be reduced, slowing down cognitive and physical responses.

Emotional and Behavioral Effects

- **Mood Disorders:** Depression, anxiety, and mood swings are prevalent following brain injury, often exacerbated by the challenges of adjusting to new limitations.

- **Personality Changes:** Changes in personality, such as increased irritability, impulsivity, or apathy, can strain relationships and social interactions.

- **Post-Traumatic Stress Disorder (PTSD):** Some individuals may experience PTSD, primarily if the brain injury resulted from a traumatic event.

Social Effects

- **Relationships:** The changes in cognitive, emotional, and physical functioning can significantly alter interpersonal relationships and social dynamics.

- **Employment:** Returning to work may be challenging, requiring adjustments in job duties or working hours, or may not be possible for some individuals.

- **Independence:** The level of independence may be reduced, with some individuals requiring assistance with daily living activities or long-term care.

Rehabilitation and Recovery

Rehabilitation efforts are tailored to the individual's needs and can include physical therapy, occupational therapy, speech and language therapy, psychological support, and cognitive rehabilitation. The goals of rehabilitation are to maximize recovery, enhance functional abilities, and improve quality of life.

The recovery trajectory varies widely; some individuals may experience significant improvements, while others may face long-term challenges. Factors influencing recovery include the severity of the injury, the individual's age, the presence of pre-existing conditions, and the timeliness and appropriateness of the rehabilitation received.

In summary, the impact of brain injury can be profound and multifaceted, affecting virtually every aspect of an individual's life. Comprehensive care and rehabilitation are essential for supporting individuals with brain injuries, facilitating recovery, and helping them adapt to changes in their abilities and lifestyles.

10.4 Exercise: 10 MCQs with Answers at the End

Test your understanding of neuropsychological disorders, the effects of brain injury, and their impact on individuals with these multiple-choice questions. Answers are provided at the end for self-assessment.

1. Which disorder is characterized by progressive memory decline and other cognitive impairments?

   - A) Parkinson's Disease

   - B) Alzheimer's Disease

   - C) Schizophrenia

   - D) Bipolar Disorder

2. A stroke results from:

   - A) Degeneration of dopamine-producing neurons

   - B) An interruption or reduction of blood supply to the brain

- C) The accumulation of amyloid-beta plaques

- D) Traumatic physical impact to the head

3. Aphasia, a disorder affecting speech and language, can result from damage to:

- A) The frontal lobe

- B) The occipital lobe

- C) The parietal lobe

- D) The temporal lobe

4. Which part of the brain are executive functions primarily associated with?

- A) Cerebellum

- B) Prefrontal Cortex

- C) Hippocampus

- D) Amygdala

5. Which neuropsychological disorder is associated with delusions, hallucinations, and disorganized speech?

- A) Major Depressive Disorder

- B) Obsessive-Compulsive Disorder

- C) Schizophrenia

- D) Autism Spectrum Disorder

6. Traumatic Brain Injury (TBI) severity is classified as:

   - A) Mild, Moderate, and Severe

   - B) Primary, Secondary, and Tertiary

   - C) Acute, Chronic, and Terminal

   - D) Type I, Type II, and Type III

7. Visual-perceptual difficulties following a brain injury are most likely to involve impairments in the:

   - A) Frontal lobe

   - B) Temporal lobe

   - C) Parietal lobe

   - D) Cerebellum

8. Which disorder is associated with the somatic marker hypothesis, essential in understanding decision-making processes?

   - A) Alzheimer's Disease

   - B) Parkinson's Disease

   - C) Schizophrenia

   - D) Autism Spectrum Disorder

9. Which is NOT a common effect of aging on cognitive functions?

   - A) Decline in episodic memory

   - B) Improvement in processing speed

   - C) Stability in semantic memory

   - D) Changes in attentional control

10. Neuroplasticity refers to:

   - A) The brain's susceptibility to neurological disorders

   - B) The brain's ability to reorganize itself by forming new neural connections

   - C) The decline in neural connections with age

   - D) The process of synaptic pruning in adulthood

Answers:

1. B) Alzheimer's Disease

2. B) An interruption or reduction of blood supply to the brain

3. D) The temporal lobe

4. B) Prefrontal Cortex

5. C) Schizophrenia

6. A) Mild, Moderate, and Severe

7. C) Parietal lobe

8. A) Alzheimer's Disease

9. B) Improvement in processing speed

10. B) The brain's ability to reorganize itself by forming new neural connections

These questions are designed to test your knowledge of neuropsychological disorders and the impact of brain injury. Reviewing your answers will help you gauge your understanding of these complex topics and identify areas for further study.

Chapter 11: Neuroimaging Techniques

11.1 An Overview of Neuroimaging

Neuroimaging is a branch of medical imaging that focuses on the brain and provides valuable insights into its structure, function, and pathology. These techniques have revolutionized neuroscience, enabling researchers and clinicians to visualize the brain in unprecedented detail, diagnose neurological and psychiatric conditions more accurately, and understand the neural bases of cognition and behavior. Neuroimaging methods can be broadly categorized into structural imaging, which provides information about the brain's anatomy, and functional imaging, which measures aspects of brain activity.

Structural Imaging Techniques

- **Computed Tomography (CT):** Uses X-rays to create detailed cross-sectional brain images. CT scans are beneficial for detecting bleeding, tumors, and structural abnormalities.

- **Magnetic Resonance Imaging (MRI):** Utilizes strong magnetic fields and radio waves to generate detailed brain images. MRI offers higher-resolution images than CT and is particularly effective for identifying abnormalities in brain tissue and structure.

Functional Imaging Techniques

- **Functional MRI (fMRI):** Measures brain activity by detecting changes in blood flow under the assumption that cerebral blood flow and neuronal activation are linked. fMRI is widely used in research to explore the brain's functional anatomy during different cognitive tasks.

- **Positron Emission Tomography (PET):** Involves injecting a radioactive tracer into the bloodstream, which is then taken up by active brain regions. PET scans are used to observe metabolic processes in the brain, aiding in the diagnosis of conditions like Alzheimer's disease.

- **Electroencephalography (EEG):** Records electrical activity along the scalp produced by firing neurons within the brain. EEG is invaluable for diagnosing epilepsy, studying sleep disorders, and researching cognitive functions due to its high temporal resolution.

- **Magnetoencephalography (MEG):** Detects the magnetic fields produced by neural activity, offering precise timing information and better spatial resolution than EEG. MEG is used to study brain function and to localize brain activity before surgery for epilepsy.

Applications of Neuroimaging

Neuroimaging has a wide range of applications, from clinical diagnosis and treatment planning to fundamental research into the workings of the human brain. In the clinical realm, neuroimaging is crucial for identifying structural abnormalities, such as tumors or brain damage from stroke, as well as for understanding functional disturbances in conditions like epilepsy, schizophrenia, and dementia. In research, neuroimaging techniques are used to explore the neural correlates of cognitive processes, such as memory, attention, and language, and to study the effects of various interventions on brain function.

Challenges and Future Directions

Despite the advances in neuroimaging, there are challenges, including the high cost of imaging technology, the need for specialized expertise, and the interpretation of complex data. Additionally, ethical considerations arise regarding using neuroimaging in predicting neurological and psychiatric conditions and understanding consciousness. Future directions in neuroimaging research aim to improve imaging techniques' resolution, speed, and affordability, develop new tracers for PET scans, and enhance data analysis methods to understand better the vast amounts of data generated.

In summary, neuroimaging techniques offer powerful tools for visualizing the structure and function of the brain, contributing to our understanding of the neural basis of health and disease. These technologies continue to evolve, promising further insights into the complexities of the human brain.

11.2 Functional MRI (fMRI)

Functional Magnetic Resonance Imaging (fMRI) is a non-invasive neuroimaging technique that measures brain activity by detecting changes associated with blood flow. This method relies on the principle of blood oxygenation level-dependent (BOLD) contrast, which reflects the increased blood flow to areas of the brain that are more active during a task or at rest. Since active neurons consume more oxygen, the local increase in oxygenated blood correlates with neuronal activity. fMRI has become a cornerstone in cognitive neuroscience and clinical neurology due to its ability to map the functional areas of the brain with high spatial resolution.

Principles of fMRI

- **BOLD Contrast:** fMRI utilizes the BOLD contrast mechanism, which is based on the magnetic properties of blood. Oxygenated and deoxygenated hemoglobin have different magnetic susceptibilities, allowing fMRI to detect changes in the ratio of oxygenated to deoxygenated blood, indirectly indicating neuronal activity.

- **Spatial and Temporal Resolution:** fMRI provides relatively high spatial resolution, on the order of 1-3 millimeters, allowing for detailed brain activity mapping. However, its temporal resolution is It is limited by the slow hemodynamic response, typically on the order of seconds, which is slower than the millisecond scale of neuronal firing.

Applications of fMRI

- **Cognitive Neuroscience:** fMRI is extensively used in cognitive neuroscience research to study the neural mechanisms underlying mental processes such as perception, memory, language, and emotion. Researchers can identify the brain regions associated with these functions by having participants perform specific tasks while undergoing fMRI scanning.

- **Brain Mapping:** Before surgical procedures for epilepsy or tumor removal, fMRI maps critical functional areas (e.g., those involved in language and motor functions) to avoid damaging these regions during surgery.

- **Clinical Diagnosis:** fMRI aids in diagnosing and evaluating neurological and psychiatric conditions by revealing functional abnormalities in the brain that may not be visible with structural imaging techniques.

- **Resting-State fMRI:** This application involves scanning the brain. At the same time, a participant is not engaged in any specific task, allowing researchers to examine the brain's functional connectivity and identify active networks at rest, such as the default mode network.

Advantages and Limitations

- **Advantages:** fMRI is non-invasive, does not involve ionizing radiation, and provides functional and anatomical information. Its high spatial resolution makes it particularly useful for mapping brain function.

- **Limitations:** The indirect measurement of neuronal activity through hemodynamic responses can be a limitation. fMRI is also sensitive to motion artifacts, and the need for participants to remain still during scanning can be challenging, especially for specific populations. The cost and accessibility of MRI technology are additional considerations.

Future Directions

Research in fMRI technology continues to focus on improving spatial and temporal resolution, developing new data analysis techniques, and integrating fMRI data with other neuroimaging modalities to provide a more comprehensive understanding of brain function. Advances in machine learning and artificial intelligence are also enhancing the ability to interpret complex fMRI datasets, opening new avenues for understanding the brain's functional architecture and its alterations in disease.

In summary, fMRI is a powerful tool for studying brain activity and has significantly advanced our understanding of the neural basis of cognition, behavior, and neuropsychological disorders. Its continued development promises to further illuminate the complexities of brain function in health and disease.

11.3 PET and EEG

Positron Emission Tomography (PET)

Positron Emission Tomography (PET) is a functional imaging technique used to observe metabolic processes in the body, including the brain. PET scans can visualize and measure changes in metabolic activity by injecting a small amount of radioactive tracers (or radioligands) into the bloodstream. In neuroimaging, PET is particularly valuable for studying brain disorders, mapping brain function, and evaluating neurodegenerative diseases.

Principles of PET

- **Radioactive Tracers:** PET imaging involves using compounds labeled with positron-emitting radioisotopes. Commonly used tracers in neuroimaging include fluorodeoxyglucose (FDG), which is taken up by active brain cells to visualize glucose metabolism.

- **Detection of Gamma Rays:** When the radioactive tracer decays, it emits positrons that collide with electrons, producing gamma rays. The PET scanner detects These gamma rays, creating a three-dimensional image of tracer concentration in the brain.

Applications of PET

- **Neurodegenerative Diseases:** PET is instrumental in diagnosing conditions like Alzheimer's by detecting amyloid plaques or tau protein tangles in the brain.

- **Brain Function:** PET can map brain activity by highlighting areas of high glucose consumption or blood flow, aiding in studying cognitive functions and the effects of various interventions.

- **Cancer Diagnosis:** Beyond neuroimaging, PET scans are widely used in oncology to detect cancerous tumors and monitor treatment efficacy.

Electroencephalography (EEG)

Electroencephalography (EEG) is a technique that records the brain's electrical activity using electrodes placed along the scalp. EEG is renowned for its excellent temporal resolution, capturing brain activity at the millisecond level, which makes it particularly suited for studying the dynamics of brain processes.

Principles of EEG

- **Electrical Activity:** EEG measures voltage fluctuations from ionic current flows within the brain's neurons. The recorded signals reflect the summation of synchronous activity of thousands or millions of neurons.

- **Waveforms:** EEG data is characterized by waveforms that vary in frequency and amplitude, which can be associated with different states of brain function, such as wakefulness, sleep, and various stages of consciousness.

Applications of EEG

- **Diagnosis of Neurological Conditions:** EEG is a cornerstone in diagnosing epilepsy, revealing characteristic patterns associated with seizures. It's also used in diagnosing sleep disorders, coma, and encephalopathies.

- **Cognitive and Behavioral Research:** Researchers use EEG to study cognitive processes such as perception, attention, and memory. Event-related potentials (ERPs), specific waveforms elicited in response to stimuli, are beneficial for this purpose.

- **Brain-Computer Interfaces (BCIs):** EEG is used in developing BCIs, which allow direct communication between the brain and external devices, beneficial for individuals with severe motor impairments.

Advantages and Limitations

- **PET:** Provides valuable insights into the brain's biochemical processes, but the cost limits its use, the need for radioactive tracers, and relatively low spatial resolution compared to MRI.

- **EEG:** Offers unmatched temporal resolution and is inexpensive and non-invasive. However, its spatial resolution is limited, and the data can be challenging to interpret due to the complexity of brain activity and the influence of non-brain sources on the signal.

In summary, PET and EEG are powerful neuroimaging techniques with unique strengths. PET excels in revealing the metabolic activity and biochemical changes in the brain, which is critical for understanding neurodegenerative diseases. At the same time, EEG's strength lies in its ability to capture the dynamic processes of brain activity, making it indispensable in clinical neurology and cognitive neuroscience.

11.4 Exercise: 10 MCQs with Answers at the End

Test your knowledge of neuroimaging techniques, including PET, EEG, and fMRI, with these multiple-choice questions. Answers are provided at the end for self-assessment.

1. What does fMRI measure to assess brain activity?

   - A) Electrical activity

   - B) Metabolic activity

   - C) Blood oxygen level-dependent (BOLD) signal

   - D) Radioactive tracer decay

2. Which neuroimaging technique uses radioactive tracers?

   - A) MRI

   - B) PET

   - C) EEG

   - D) CT

3. EEG is beneficial for diagnosing:

   - A) Alzheimer's disease

   - B) Epilepsy

   - C) Brain tumors

   - D) Stroke

4. The primary advantage of PET scans in neuroimaging is their ability to:

   - A) Provide high-resolution structural images

   - B) Measure electrical activity in the brain

   - C) Visualize metabolic processes and biochemical activity

   - D) Directly observe neuronal firing

5. What aspect of brain function is EEG best at measuring?

   - A) Brain structure

   - B) Blood flow

   - C) Temporal dynamics of brain activity

- D) Metabolic activity

6. Which of the following is NOT a typical application of fMRI?

   - A) Mapping brain function during cognitive tasks

- B) Diagnosing neurodegenerative diseases by detecting amyloid plaques

   - C) Studying the effects of drugs on brain activity

   - D) Observing changes in brain activity over time

7. The spatial resolution of EEG is:

   - A) High

   - B) Moderate

   - C) Low

   - D) Variable

8. PET scans can be particularly useful in diagnosing which condition by detecting amyloid plaques.

   - A) Parkinson's Disease

   - B) Epilepsy

   - C) Alzheimer's Disease

   - D) Multiple Sclerosis

9. The BOLD signal in fMRI reflects changes in:

   - A) Neuronal action potentials

   - B) Blood oxygenation levels

   - C) Glucose metabolism

   - D) Calcium ion concentration

10. Which neuroimaging technique is known for its excellent temporal resolution?

   - A) MRI

   - B) PET

   - C) EEG

   - D) CT

Answers:

1. C) Blood oxygen level-dependent (BOLD) signal

2. B) PET

3. B) Epilepsy

4. C) Visualize metabolic processes and biochemical activity

5. C) Temporal dynamics of brain activity

6. B) Diagnosing neurodegenerative diseases by detecting amyloid plaques

7. C) Low

8. C) Alzheimer's Disease

9. B) Blood oxygenation levels

10. C) EEG

These questions are designed to assess your understanding of various neuroimaging techniques and their applications, highlighting each method's unique capabilities and limitations in studying brain structure and function. Reviewing your answers can help reinforce your neuroimaging knowledge and its importance in research and clinical settings.

Chapter 12: Cognitive Enhancement

12.1 Techniques for Cognitive Improvement

Cognitive enhancement refers to using various techniques, strategies, and interventions to improve cognitive functions such as memory, attention, executive functions, and problem-solving skills. Interest in cognitive enhancement spans from clinical applications, aiming to assist individuals with cognitive impairments, to the broader public seeking to optimize mental performance for academic, professional, or personal reasons. This section explores several evidence-based techniques and interventions for cognitive improvement.

Physical Exercise

- Regular physical activity is one of the most effective means of enhancing cognitive function across the lifespan. Exercise promotes neurogenesis (the growth of new neurons), improves brain plasticity, and increases cerebral blood flow. It has been linked to attention, memory, executive functions, and mood improvements.

Nutrition and Diet

- A balanced diet rich in omega-3 fatty acids, antioxidants, vitamins, and minerals supports brain health and cognitive function. Diets such as the Mediterranean diet, which emphasizes fruits, vegetables, whole grains, and healthy fats, have been associated with a lower risk of cognitive decline and dementia.

Cognitive Training

- Cognitive training programs, including computer-based exercises designed to target specific cognitive domains, can lead to improvements in those areas. While transferring these gains to everyday cognitive functioning is still a research subject, some studies suggest benefits in memory, attention, and problem-solving skills.

Mindfulness and Meditation

- Mindfulness meditation practices have been shown to improve attention, working memory, executive functioning, and emotional regulation. Regular meditation can also reduce stress and anxiety, which can indirectly benefit cognitive function.

Sleep Hygiene

- Adequate sleep is crucial for cognitive processes, including memory consolidation, attention, and executive functions. Practices that promote good sleep hygiene, such as maintaining a consistent sleep schedule and creating a comfortable sleep environment, can enhance cognitive performance and overall mental health.

Social Engagement

- Active social engagement and maintaining a supportive social network have been associated with better cognitive function and a lower risk of cognitive decline. Social interactions can stimulate cognitive processes and contribute to emotional well-being.

Lifelong Learning

- Engaging in lifelong learning activities, such as taking courses, learning a new language, or acquiring new skills, can promote cognitive health by providing mental stimulation and building cognitive reserve.

Pharmacological Interventions

Certain medications and supplements are marketed for cognitive enhancement, but their effectiveness and safety can vary. Some substances, such as caffeine and nicotine, have known short-term mental enhancement effects, but long-term use or misuse can have negative health consequences. Always consult healthcare professionals before starting any pharmacological interventions for cognitive enhancement.

Neuromodulation Techniques

- Emerging technologies such as transcranial direct current stimulation (tDCS) and transcranial magnetic stimulation (TMS) offer potential avenues for cognitive enhancement by modulating neural activity. However, these approaches are currently more common in research settings and clinical treatment for specific conditions rather than widespread cognitive enhancement use.

Cognitive enhancement encompasses various techniques and interventions to improve cognitive function. While some strategies have strong evidence supporting their effectiveness, the field is rapidly evolving, with ongoing research into new and innovative approaches to enhancing cognitive abilities.

12.2 The Ethics of Cognitive Enhancement

Cognitive enhancement raises significant ethical considerations, mainly through pharmacological means or emerging technologies. These concerns revolve around fairness, coercion, the nature of human achievement, and the potential long-term impacts on society. As cognitive enhancement becomes more prevalent and accessible, it is crucial to address these ethical issues to guide responsible use and policy development.

Fairness and Equality

- **Access:** One of the primary ethical concerns is the unequal access to cognitive enhancement technologies and drugs. This inequality could exacerbate existing social disparities, creating further advantages for those who can afford or have access to these interventions.

- **Competitive Environments:** In academic and professional settings, the use of cognitive enhancers could pressure individuals to use these substances to remain competitive, potentially leading to an arms race of enhancement.

Coercion and Autonomy

- **Social and Institutional Pressure:** There is concern that widespread acceptance of cognitive enhancement could lead to direct or indirect coercion, where individuals feel compelled to use these methods to meet societal or professional expectations.

- **Informed Consent:** The autonomy of individuals to make informed decisions about cognitive enhancement is crucial, especially considering the potential risks and side effects of pharmacological agents.

Safety and Long-term Effects

- **Health Risks:** The long-term health impacts of cognitive enhancement drugs and technologies are not fully understood. The use of substances not approved for cognitive enhancement or "off-label" use of prescription medications carries risks.

- **Neurological Development:** There are particular concerns about using cognitive enhancers in children and adolescents whose brains are still developing. The long-term effects on neural development and psychological well-being are unknown.

Identity and Human Achievement

- **Authenticity:** Some argue that cognitive enhancement could undermine the authenticity of personal achievements, questioning whether successes result from individual effort or the effect of enhancement.

- **Human Nature:** There are philosophical debates about whether cognitive enhancement aligns with or deviates from human nature and whether it represents an evolutionary step or a departure from what it means to be human.

Regulation and Policy Development

- **Legal and Regulatory Frameworks:** The development of legal and regulatory frameworks that balance the potential benefits of cognitive enhancement with ethical concerns and health risks is essential. This includes policies on using, distributing, and marketing cognitive enhancers.

- **Research and Transparency:** Encouraging transparent and ethical research into the efficacy and safety of cognitive enhancement methods can inform policy decisions and public understanding.

Public Discourse and Education

- Engaging the public in discourse about the ethical implications of cognitive enhancement and providing education on the risks and benefits can foster informed decision-making and ethical use.

In summary, the ethics of cognitive enhancement encompasses a wide array of considerations, from fairness and autonomy to the potential impacts on human nature and society. Addressing these ethical issues requires a multidisciplinary approach involving ethicists, scientists, policymakers, and the public to navigate the complexities of enhancing cognitive function responsibly.

12.3 Future Directions in Cognitive Enhancement

The field of cognitive enhancement is rapidly evolving, with advances in neuroscience, technology, and pharmacology promising new avenues for enhancing brain function. Future directions in cognitive enhancement will likely focus on personalized approaches, integration of various Enhancement strategies, ethical considerations, and developing safer, more effective interventions. Here are some potential future trends and areas of focus:

Personalized Cognitive Enhancement

- Advances in genomics and neuroimaging may enable more personalized approaches to cognitive enhancement, tailoring interventions to an individual's genetic makeup, brain structure, and specific cognitive profiles. This could optimize the effectiveness of interventions while minimizing side effects.

Combining Pharmacological and Non-Pharmacological Approaches

- There is growing interest in combining different cognitive enhancement strategies, such as pharmacological agents, mental training, physical exercise, and dietary interventions. This multimodal approach could synergize benefits and address cognitive function more holistically.

Advancements in Neurotechnology

- Emerging neurotechnologies, including brain-computer interfaces (BCIs), transcranial magnetic stimulation (TMS), and transcranial direct current stimulation (tDCS), offer novel ways to enhance cognitive function directly by modulating brain activity. Ongoing research aims to improve the efficacy, safety, and accessibility of these technologies.

- Wearable neurotechnology and mobile applications that support cognitive training and mindfulness practices may become more integrated into daily life, offering accessible ways to enhance cognitive function.

Ethical Frameworks and Regulation

- As cognitive enhancement technologies and pharmacological agents develop, there will be an increasing need for ethical frameworks and regulatory policies that address concerns about fairness, autonomy, and the long-term impacts on individuals and society. This includes guidelines for cognitive enhancers in healthy individuals, children, and vulnerable populations.

Enhancing Cognitive Aging

- With the global population aging, there is significant interest in interventions that support cognitive health in older adults. Research may focus on preventing cognitive decline, enhancing cognitive reserve, and developing interventions that specifically address age-related changes in brain function.

Neuroplasticity and Lifelong Learning

- Understanding the mechanisms underlying neuroplasticity could lead to new strategies for enhancing cognitive function across the lifespan. This includes interventions that promote brain plasticity through environmental enrichment, learning new skills, and engaging in intellectually stimulating activities.

Public Education and Awareness

- As cognitive enhancement becomes more prevalent, there will be a need for public education campaigns to inform individuals about the potential benefits, risks, and ethical considerations. This can empower individuals to make informed decisions about cognitive enhancement interventions.

Global Collaboration and Research

- Collaborative international research efforts can accelerate the development of effective cognitive enhancement interventions and address global disparities in access to these technologies and treatments.

In summary, the future of cognitive enhancement is poised for significant advancements, potentially improving cognitive function, supporting healthy aging, and enhancing quality of life. However, these developments must be guided by rigorous scientific research, ethical considerations, and equitable access to ensure they benefit individuals and society.

12.4 Exercise: 10 MCQs with Answers at the End

Test your knowledge of cognitive enhancement, including techniques, ethical considerations, and future directions, with these multiple-choice questions. Answers are provided at the end for self-assessment.

1. Which is an evidence-based method for cognitive enhancement?

  - A) Prolonged sleep deprivation

  - B) Physical exercise

- C) High sugar diet

- D) Passive television watching

2. Personalized cognitive enhancement may benefit from advancements in:

- A) Astrology

- B) Genomics

- C) Paleontology

- D) Mythology

3. Which neurotechnology is used for direct modulation of brain activity?

- A) EEG

- B) TMS

- C) PET

- D) MRI

4. An ethical concern associated with cognitive enhancement is:

- A) Improved physical health

- B) Unequal access

- C) Decreased productivity

- D) Enhanced natural beauty

5. Combining pharmacological agents with ______________ represents a multimodal approach to cognitive enhancement.

- A) Cognitive training

- B) Increased screen time

- C) Social isolation

- D) Sedentary lifestyle

6. The use of mobile applications for cognitive training is an example of:

- A) Wearable neurotechnology

- B) Passive entertainment

- C) Traditional education methods

- D) Invasive surgery

7. Future cognitive enhancement technologies might focus on:

- A) Reducing neuroplasticity

- B) Personalized interventions based on genetic and brain profiles

- C) Eliminating the need for sleep

- D) Increasing reliance on fossil fuels

8. Regular ___________ is crucial for maintaining cognitive function in older adults.

   - A) Alcohol consumption

   - B) Physical exercise

   - C) Exposure to pollutants

   - D) High-stress environments

9. Ethical frameworks for cognitive enhancement are needed to address:

   - A) The benefits of universal enhancement

   - B) Fairness and the potential for coercion

   - C) The importance of eliminating all challenges

   - D) Encouraging a sedentary lifestyle

10. Collaborative international research in cognitive enhancement aims to:

   - A) Slow scientific progress

   - B) Create a monopoly on technology

   - C) Accelerate development and address global disparities

   - D) Focus solely on high-income countries

Answers:

1. B) Physical exercise

2. B) Genomics

3. B) TMS

4. B) Unequal access

5. A) Cognitive training

6. A) Wearable neurotechnology

7. B) Personalized interventions based on genetic and brain profiles

8. B) Physical exercise

9. B) Fairness and the potential for coercion

10. C) Accelerate development and address global disparities

These questions are designed to assess your understanding of the critical concepts related to cognitive enhancement, including current practices, technological advancements, ethical considerations, and the potential for future developments in the field. Reviewing your answers can help reinforce your knowledge and identify areas for further exploration.

Chapter 13: Consciousness and Cognition

13.1 Theories of Consciousness

Consciousness, the state of being aware of and able to think about one's existence, sensations, thoughts, and environment, remains one of psychology and neuroscience's most intriguing subjects. It encompasses the experiences of perception, thought, emotion, self-awareness, and intentionality. Several theories attempt to explain the nature of consciousness and its mechanisms:

Global Workspace Theory (GWT)

- Proposed by Bernard Baars, GWT suggests that consciousness arises as a function of the global availability of information across different neural systems. According to this theory, conscious experience results from information being broadcasted in a worldwide workspace—a network of interconnected neurons that can access and process information from various sensory inputs and cognitive processes.

Integrated Information Theory (IIT)

- Developed by Giulio Tononi, IIT posits that consciousness corresponds to the level of information integration within a system. The theory asserts that a system is conscious to the extent that it contains a high degree of integrated information, which cannot be reduced to separate components. IIT attempts to quantify consciousness through a measure called Φ (phi), representing the amount of integrated information.

Higher-Order Theories (HOTs)

- Higher-order theories, including Higher-Order Thought (HOT) theory, argue that consciousness arises when a mental state is the object of another mental state. In other words, a thought or perception becomes conscious only when it is the subject of another idea. HOTs distinguish between phenomenal consciousness (the subjective experience of sensations and perceptions) and access consciousness (the processing of information for cognitive usage).

Predictive Processing Framework

- This framework suggests that the brain constantly generates and updates predictions about sensory inputs based on past experiences. Consciousness, in this view, emerges from the brain's attempts to minimize the error between its predictions and the actual sensory input. This ongoing prediction and error correction process is believed to give rise to conscious experience.

Panpsychism

- Panpsychism is a philosophical view positing that consciousness is a fundamental and ubiquitous feature of the physical world. According to this perspective, even elementary particles exhibit primitive forms of consciousness, suggesting that consciousness is not exclusive to complex brains but is inherent in all matter to some degree.

Quantum Theories of Consciousness

- Some theorists propose that quantum mechanics plays a crucial role in consciousness. Theories like Roger Penrose's and Stuart Hameroff's Orchestrated Objective Reduction (Orch-OR) suggest that quantum processes in the brain's microtubules could generate conscious experience. These theories are highly speculative and remain controversial within the scientific community.

Each of these theories offers a unique perspective on consciousness, reflecting this phenomenon's complexity and multifaceted nature. Despite the diversity of views, a common goal among researchers is to understand how subjective experiences arise from neural processes and how consciousness impacts cognition and behavior. The study of consciousness continues to challenge our understanding of the mind, bridging psychology, neuroscience, philosophy, and even quantum physics.

13.2 States of Consciousness

States of consciousness refer to the different levels of awareness of the external world and one's internal thoughts and feelings. These states range from full alertness and wakefulness to various altered states, such as sleep, dreaming, hypnotic states, meditative states, and the effects of psychoactive drugs. Understanding these states provides insights into how consciousness operates and its variations across different conditions.

Wakefulness

- This is the state of consciousness in which individuals are fully aware and responsive to external stimuli. It is characterized by cognitive functions such as perception, thinking, decision-making, and problem-solving.

Sleep

- Sleep is a naturally recurring state of altered consciousness, relatively reduced sensory activity, and inhibition of nearly all voluntary muscles. It is distinguished into two main types: rapid eye movement (REM) sleep and non-REM (NREM) sleep, each with distinct brain activity patterns. REM sleep is associated with vivid dreaming, while NREM sleep is divided into stages of increasing depth of sleep.

Dreaming

- Dreaming occurs primarily during REM sleep, though it can happen in other sleep stages. Dreams are images, ideas, emotions, and sensations that occur involuntarily in the mind. The function and significance of dreaming in cognition and emotional processing are subjects of ongoing research.

Hypnosis

- Hypnosis is a state of focused attention, increased suggestibility, and vivid fantasies. People in a hypnotic state often feel calm and relaxed and may be more open to suggestions. Hypnosis is used therapeutically to manage pain, reduce stress, and treat various psychological disorders.

Meditation

- Meditation involves practices that focus or redirect thoughts to achieve a mentally clear, emotionally calm, and stable state. Different forms of meditation can induce changes in consciousness, leading to enhanced self-awareness, reduced stress, and deeper states of relaxation.

Psychoactive Drugs

- Psychoactive drugs, including stimulants, depressants, hallucinogens, and opioids, can significantly alter consciousness. These substances affect brain chemistry and can change perception, mood, consciousness, and behavior. The effects vary widely depending on the type of drug, dosage, and individual differences.

Altered States of Consciousness

- Altered states of consciousness can be induced by various means, including sensory deprivation, sleep deprivation, fasting, and the use of psychoactive substances. Changes in perception, thought processes, self-awareness, or emotions characterize these states.

Function and Importance

- Studying different states of consciousness contributes to our understanding of the human mind, including the mechanisms underlying consciousness, the brain's adaptability, and various states' psychological and physiological functions. Additionally, exploring altered states of consciousness can offer insights into creativity, problem-solving, and the therapeutic potential of manipulating consciousness.

In summary, states of consciousness encompass a broad spectrum of experiences, from the alertness of wakefulness to the altered perceptions of psychoactive drug use. Research into these states enriches our understanding of consciousness and has practical implications for health, well-being, and the treatment of psychological disorders.

13.3 The Unconscious Mind

The unconscious mind plays a central role in various psychological theories, particularly in psychoanalytic theory, where it is considered a reservoir of feelings, thoughts, urges, and memories outside our conscious awareness. The unconscious mind influences behavior and decision-making, often in ways individuals are unaware of. Modern psychology and neuroscience have expanded our understanding of unconscious processes, recognizing that much cognitive processing occurs outside conscious awareness.

Psychoanalytic Perspective

- Sigmund Freud, the founder of psychoanalysis, conceptualized the unconscious as a storehouse of repressed desires, traumatic memories, and unresolved conflicts. He suggested that these unconscious elements could manifest in dreams, slips of the tongue ("Freudian slips"), and neuroses. Freud distinguished between the preconscious (thoughts that are not conscious but can become aware) and the unconscious mind.

Cognitive Psychology Perspective

- Cognitive psychologists approach the unconscious from the information processing perspective, focusing on how people automatically process vast amounts of information without conscious awareness. This includes perceptions, memories, and attitudes that influence thoughts and behaviors. Cognitive psychology studies phenomena such as priming, where exposure to a stimulus affects the response to a subsequent stimulus without the individual being aware of the influence.

The Role of the Unconscious in Decision-Making

- Research suggests that the unconscious mind plays a significant role in decision-making. For complex decisions, the "deliberation-without-attention" effect indicates that people often make better choices after distraction, allowing their unconscious to process the information, compared to when they consciously deliberate on the options.

Neuroscience and the Unconscious

- Neuroscience research has identified neural correlates of unconscious processes, including the brain mechanisms involved in automatic behaviors, subliminal perception, and implicit memory. Functional magnetic resonance imaging (fMRI) and electroencephalography (EEG) have allowed scientists to study the brain activity associated with unconscious processing.

The Adaptive Unconscious

- Psychologist Timothy D. Wilson introduced the concept of the adaptive unconscious, which he describes as the mental processes that automatically affect emotions, preferences, and behaviors. These processes are adaptive, as they efficiently handle routine tasks and make rapid judgments, freeing up the conscious mind for more complex problems.

Implicit Biases

- The unconscious mind is also the source of implicit biases—unconscious attitudes or stereotypes that unconsciously affect understanding, actions, and decisions. These biases can influence social behavior and perceptions, often in ways that conflict with conscious beliefs about equality and fairness.

Therapeutic Approaches

- Various therapeutic approaches aim to bring unconscious material into consciousness, facilitating healing and personal growth. Techniques include psychoanalysis, dream analysis, and certain forms of psychotherapy that explore unconscious motivations and conflicts.

In summary, the unconscious mind encompasses vast cognitive processes outside of conscious awareness, influencing thoughts, feelings, and behaviors. Understanding the unconscious mind requires a multidisciplinary approach, combining insights from psychoanalysis, cognitive psychology, and neuroscience. This exploration deepens our understanding of human cognition and behavior and has practical implications for therapy, decision-making, and addressing implicit biases.

13.4 Exercise: 10 MCQs with Answers at the End

Test your understanding of theories of consciousness, states of consciousness, the unconscious mind, and related concepts with these multiple-choice questions. Answers are provided at the end for self-assessment.

1. Who is most closely associated with the development of psychoanalytic theory and the concept of the unconscious mind?

 - A) Jean Piaget

 - B) Sigmund Freud

 - C) B.F. Skinner

 - D) Carl Rogers

2. The Global Workspace Theory of consciousness suggests that consciousness arises from:

   - A) The accumulation of sensory experiences

   - B) The integration of information across different neural systems

   - C) The functioning of the brain's right hemisphere

   - D) Quantum processes within neurons

3. Which state of consciousness is characterized by rapid eye movement and vivid dreaming?

   - A) Deep sleep

   - B) Hypnosis

   - C) REM sleep

   - D) Meditation

4. The "deliberation-without-attention" effect demonstrates that complex decisions can sometimes be improved by:

   - A) Focusing intensely on the problem

   - B) Allowing the unconscious mind to process information

   - C) Seeking advice from others

   - D) Using logical reasoning only

5. Which technique measures brain activity by detecting changes associated with blood flow and is used to study brain function?

- A) PET

- B) EEG

- C) fMRI

- D) TMS

6. Implicit biases are examples of:

- A) Conscious attitudes that align with one's behavior

- B) Unconscious attitudes that influence understanding and actions

- C) Deliberate decisions to act in a certain way

- D) Memories that can be easily recalled

7. Integrated Information Theory (IIT) of consciousness proposes that consciousness corresponds to:

- A) The level of alertness of an individual

- B) The amount of integrated information within a system

- C) The number of active synapses in the brain

- D) The frequency of neural oscillations

8. Which is NOT a typical application of EEG?

 - A) Diagnosing epilepsy

 - B) Studying sleep disorders

 - C) Mapping brain function during surgery

 - D) Observing metabolic processes in the brain

9. Which state of consciousness is meditation primarily associated with?

 - A) Altered state of consciousness

 - B) Unconsciousness

 - C) Subconsciousness

 - D) Preconsciousness

10. Higher-order theories (HOTs) of consciousness argue that a thought or perception becomes conscious when it is:

 - A) Associated with a strong emotional response

 - B) The subject of another thought

 - C) Processed by the left hemisphere of the brain

 - D) Stored in long-term memory

Answers:

1. B) Sigmund Freud

2. B) The integration of information across different neural systems

3. C) REM sleep

4. B) Allowing the unconscious mind to process information

5. C) fMRI

6. B) Unconscious attitudes that influence understanding and actions

7. B) The amount of integrated information within a system

8. D) Observing metabolic processes in the brain

9. A) Altered state of consciousness

10. B) The subject of another thought

These questions assess your knowledge of consciousness, unconscious processes, and the various theories and states associated with them, providing a comprehensive overview of these complex topics in cognitive science.

Chapter 14: Learning and Behavior

14.1 Principles of Learning

Learning is a fundamental process that changes behavior, skills, knowledge, or preferences based on experiences. Understanding learning principles is essential for educators, psychologists, and anyone interested in behavior change. These principles, derived from decades of psychological research, provide insights into how learning occurs and how it can be optimized.

Classical Conditioning

- **Association:** Learning involves forming associations between stimuli. Classical conditioning, demonstrated by Ivan Pavlov, shows how a neutral stimulus can acquire the capacity to elicit a response when paired with a stimulus that naturally evokes that response.

- **Generalization and Discrimination:** Generalization occurs when stimuli similar to the conditioned stimulus elicit the conditioned response. Discrimination involves the ability to differentiate between the conditioned stimulus and other stimuli.

Operant Conditioning

- **Reinforcement and Punishment:** B.F. Skinner's research on operant conditioning emphasized the role of consequences in learning. Positive reinforcement increases the likelihood of a behavior by adding a desirable outcome, while negative reinforcement increases behaviors by removing an aversive stimulus. Punishment, conversely, decreases the likelihood of a behavior.

- **Schedules of Reinforcement:** The timing and frequency of reinforcement affect the rate and strength of learning. Fixed and variable schedules, both ratio (based on the number of responses) and interval (based on the time elapsed) affect behavior differently.

Observational Learning

- **Modeling:** Albert Bandura's work demonstrated that individuals could learn new behaviors by observing and imitating others. Factors influencing observational learning include the model's characteristics, the observer's ability to reproduce the behavior, and the observer's motivation.

- **Vicarious Reinforcement:** Seeing a model rewarded for a behavior increases the likelihood of the observer engaging in that behavior, while seeing a model punished decreases that likelihood.

Cognitive Learning

- **Information Processing:** Learning involves processing information through attention, encoding, storage, and retrieval. Effective learning strategies, such as elaborative rehearsal, mnemonics, and spaced repetition, enhance these processes.

- **Problem-Solving and Insight:** Learning is not always a gradual process but can occur suddenly through insight, as demonstrated in Wolfgang Köhler's research with chimpanzees. Problem-solving skills develop through both instruction and exploratory learning.

Motivation and Learning

- **Intrinsic and Extrinsic Motivation:** Intrinsic motivation arises from the inherent pleasure or interest in the learning activity, while external rewards or pressures drive extrinsic motivation. Both types of motivation significantly impact learning engagement and outcomes.

- **Goal Setting and Self-Efficacy:** Setting achievable goals and believing in one's ability to accomplish those goals (self-efficacy) are crucial for sustained learning and behavior change.

Learning Environments

- **Social and Cultural Contexts:** Learning is influenced by the social and cultural contexts in which it occurs. Social interactions, cultural practices, and language all shape learning processes and outcomes.

- **Feedback and Error Correction:** Timely and specific feedback is essential for learning. Effective feedback helps learners correct errors, refine skills, and better understand the subject matter.

In summary, learning principles encompass various phenomena, from classical and operant conditioning to observational learning, cognitive processes, and the impact of motivation and social contexts on learning. These principles highlight the complexity of learning and provide valuable guidelines for teaching, behavior modification, and self-improvement.

14.2 Conditioning and Learning

Conditioning is a fundamental concept in learning, encompassing how associations between stimuli and responses are formed and modified. The two primary types of conditioning, classical and operant conditioning, offer insight into how involuntary and voluntary behaviors are acquired and changed over time.

Classical Conditioning (Pavlovian Conditioning)

Classical conditioning involves learning to associate an initially neutral stimulus with a stimulus that naturally evokes a response, leading to the neutral stimulus triggering a similar response when presented alone. This form of learning demonstrates how environmental cues can elicit conditioned responses through association.

- **Unconditioned Stimulus (US):** A stimulus that naturally and automatically triggers a response without prior learning (e.g., food causing salivation in dogs).

- **Unconditioned Response (UR):** The natural response to the unconditioned stimulus (e.g., salivation in response to food).

- **Conditioned Stimulus (CS):** A previously neutral stimulus that eventually triggers a conditioned response after becoming associated with the unconditioned stimulus.

- **Conditioned Response (CR):** The learned response to the previously neutral, now conditioned, stimulus (e.g., salivation in response to a bell associated with food).

Operant Conditioning (Instrumental Conditioning)

Operant conditioning involves learning to associate behaviors with their consequences. Through reinforcement and punishment, behaviors can be encouraged or discouraged, illustrating how voluntary actions are shaped by their outcomes.

- **Reinforcement:** Increases the likelihood of a behavior being repeated. Positive reinforcement introduces a pleasant stimulus (e.g., praise), while negative reinforcement removes an unpleasant stimulus (e.g., turning off an annoying sound).

- **Punishment:** Decreases the likelihood of a behavior being repeated. Positive punishment introduces an unpleasant stimulus (e.g., a scolding), while negative punishment removes a pleasant stimulus (e.g., taking away a toy).

- **Schedules of Reinforcement:** The pattern and frequency of reinforcement affect the speed and strength of learning. Fixed-ratio, variable-ratio, fixed-interval, and variable-interval schedules each produce distinct response patterns.

Factors Influencing Conditioning

- **Timing:** The temporal relationship between stimuli or between behavior and its consequences significantly affects learning. In classical conditioning, the conditioned stimulus must closely precede The unconditioned stimulus. In operant conditioning, consequences must follow the behavior promptly.

- **Intensity:** The strength of the stimulus or the magnitude of the reinforcement or punishment can influence the speed and durability of learning.

- **Consistency:** Consistent association between stimuli or between behavior and consequences is crucial for effective conditioning.

- **Biological Predispositions:** Innate predispositions can facilitate or inhibit learning-specific associations, indicating that not all stimuli are equally effective as conditioned stimuli or reinforcers.

Applications of Conditioning

Conditioning principles are applied in various fields, including education, psychology, animal training, and behavior therapy. For example, classical conditioning principles underlie exposure therapy for phobias, while operant conditioning techniques are used in behavior modification programs and skill training.

In summary, conditioning and learning theories provide potent frameworks for understanding how behaviors are acquired, maintained, or modified. These principles illuminate fundamental aspects of human and animal behavior and offer practical strategies for promoting beneficial behaviors and reducing undesirable ones.

14.3 Cognitive Approaches to Learning

Cognitive approaches to learning focus on the mental processes involved in acquiring knowledge and understanding through thought, experience, and the senses. Unlike behaviorism, which emphasizes observable behaviors and their responses to stimuli, cognitive theories consider the mind's inner workings, understanding learning as an active, constructive process. This perspective highlights how individuals interpret information, solve problems, and apply what they've learned to new situations.

Information Processing Model

- The Information Processing Model likens the human mind to a computer, emphasizing how information is taken in (encoded), stored, and retrieved. It outlines several stages of memory, including sensory, short-term (working), and long-term memory, detailing how information is filtered, processed, and retained.

- **Strategies for Enhancing Memory:** Cognitive approaches suggest methods to improve learning and memory, such as chunking, mnemonics, rehearsal techniques, and elaborative encoding, which involves making meaningful connections between new information and existing knowledge.

Metacognition

- Metacognition refers to an individual's awareness and understanding of their thought processes. It involves self-regulation strategies for planning, monitoring, and evaluating one's learning and problem-solving methods. Teaching learners to be metacognitively aware can significantly improve their ability to learn effectively and adaptively apply strategies in various contexts.

Constructivism

- Constructivism posits that learners construct their understanding and knowledge of the world through experiencing things and reflecting on those experiences. It emphasizes the importance of active engagement, problem-solving, and the application of knowledge in real-world contexts.

- **Social Constructivism:** Vygotsky's theory emphasizes the social context of learning, suggesting that knowledge is constructed through interactions with others and cultural tools that shape cognitive development.

Schema Theory

- Schema theory suggests that all knowledge is organized into units (schemas), mental structures representing some aspect of the world. Learning involves assimilating new information into existing schemas and accommodating schemas to incorporate further details. This theory highlights the importance of background knowledge and information organization in learning.

Problem-Based Learning (PBL)

- Problem-Based Learning is an educational approach that uses complex, real-world problems as the context for students to develop problem-solving skills, acquire new knowledge, and learn to work collaboratively. PBL emphasizes learner autonomy and the application of knowledge, consistent with constructivist principles.

Cognitive Load Theory

- Cognitive Load Theory focuses on the amount of information that working memory can hold at one time and how instructional design can be optimized to manage cognitive load. It distinguishes between intrinsic, extraneous, and germane cognitive load, suggesting strategies to reduce cognitive overload and enhance learning.

Situated Learning

- Situated Learning theory proposes that learning occurs through participation in social and cultural contexts, emphasizing the importance of authentic contexts in which learners engage in meaningful activities and interact with expert practitioners.

Cognitive approaches to learning have significantly influenced educational practices, instructional design, and our understanding of how learning occurs. Acknowledging the complexity of mental processes, these theories offer nuanced insights into effective teaching and learning strategies that foster deep knowledge, critical thinking, and lifelong learning skills.

14.4 Exercise: 10 MCQs with Answers at the End

Test your knowledge of the principles of learning, conditioning, cognitive approaches to education, and related concepts with these multiple-choice questions. Answers are provided at the end for self-assessment.

1. What does classical conditioning primarily involve?

   - A) Rewards and punishments

   - B) Associations between stimuli

   - C) Cognitive problem-solving

   - D) Social learning through observation

2. Operant conditioning is best described as:

   - A) Learning through association between two stimuli

   - B) Learning based on the consequences of behavior

   - C) Learning by observing and imitating others

   - D) Learning that occurs without any external rewards

3. Which concept is a critical component of the Information Processing Model?

   - A) Classical conditioning

   - B) Operant conditioning

   - C) Working memory

   - D) Social learning

4. Metacognition involves:

   - A) The unconscious mind

   - B) Awareness and understanding of one's thought processes

   - C) The physical structure of the brain

   - D) Classical conditioning processes

5. Constructivism emphasizes learning as:

   - A) A passive process of absorbing information

   - B) An active process of constructing knowledge

   - C) A series of conditioned responses

   - D) Dependent solely on genetic factors

6. The use of mnemonics is an example of a strategy to enhance:

   - A) Sensory memory

   - B) Long-term memory

   - C) Classical conditioning

  - D) Operant conditioning

7. Schema theory suggests that:

   - A) All knowledge is innate

   - B) Knowledge is organized into units or schemas

   - C) Learning occurs through punishments only

   - D) Social interactions inhibit learning

8. In Vygotsky's theory, the zone of proximal development is:

   - A) The difference between what learners can do without help and what they can achieve with guidance

   - B) A state of cognitive overload

   - C) The final stage of cognitive development

   - D) The area of the brain responsible for memory

9. Cognitive Load Theory is concerned with:

   - A) The effects of punishment on learning

   - B) Managing the amount of information processed by working memory

   - C) The role of the unconscious mind in learning

   - D) The development of conditioned responses

10. What is the principle of Problem-Based Learning (PBL)?

   - A) Learning is enhanced by passive observation

   - B) Learning occurs in isolation from real-world contexts

   - C) Learning is driven by solving real-world problems

   - D) Knowledge is transmitted from teacher to student without active engagement

Answers:

1. B) Associations between stimuli

2. B) Learning based on the consequences of behavior

3. C) Working memory

4. B) Awareness and understanding of one's thought processes

5. B) An active process of constructing knowledge

6. B) Long-term memory

7. B) Knowledge is organized into units or schemas

8. A) The difference between what learners can do without help and what they can achieve with guidance

9. B) Managing the amount of information processed by working memory

10. C) Learning is driven by solving real-world problems

These questions are designed to assess your understanding of various learning theories and approaches, highlighting key concepts and methods in the study of learning and behavior. Reviewing your answers can help reinforce your knowledge and identify areas for further exploration.

Chapter 15: Future Directions in Cognitive Neuroscience

15.1 Emerging Technologies in Brain Science

Cognitive neuroscience is at the forefront of exploring the complexities of the brain and its relation to behavior and mental processes. Advancements in technology are rapidly transforming the field, enabling researchers to delve deeper into the brain's workings and opening up new possibilities for understanding cognition and treating neurological disorders. Here are several emerging technologies that are shaping the future of brain science.

Optogenetics

- Optogenetics is a technique that uses light to control neurons genetically modified to express light-sensitive ion channels. It allows precise manipulation of neuronal activity, enabling researchers to study the function of specific brain circuits in real-time and understand how changes in these circuits affect behavior and cognitive processes.

Brain-Computer Interfaces (BCIs)

- BCIs create direct pathways between the brain and external devices, bypassing traditional neuromuscular routes. This technology has profound implications for restoring function to individuals with paralysis, enhancing cognitive abilities, and exploring new forms of communication. BCIs are also used to study the neural basis of consciousness and decision-making.

High-Density Electroencephalography (HD-EEG)

- HD-EEG involves recording brain activity with scalp electrodes using a much higher density of sensors than traditional EEG. This improvement in spatial resolution allows for more precise localization of brain activity and a better understanding of the temporal dynamics of cognitive processes.

Closed-Loop Stimulation

- Closed-loop stimulation systems monitor brain activity in real-time and deliver targeted electrical or magnetic interventions when specific patterns are detected. This approach is promising for treating conditions like epilepsy and depression, as it can modulate neural activity in a highly personalized and adaptive manner.

Single-Cell Transcriptomics and Genomics: Advances in single-cell sequencing technologies allow researchers to examine the gene expression profiles of individual neurons, providing insights into the cellular diversity of the brain and the molecular underpinnings of neural development, function, and disorders.

Advanced Neuroimaging Techniques

- Techniques such as 7 Tesla (7T) MRI and beyond offer unprecedented resolution for imaging the brain, revealing detailed anatomical structures and enabling the study of microscale processes that underlie cognitive functions. Functional neuroimaging is also advancing, with new methods for assessing connectivity and metabolic activity in the brain.

Neuroinformatics and Big Data

- The explosion of data generated by neuroscientific research requires sophisticated computational tools for analysis, visualization, and modeling. Neuroinformatics combines computational neuroscience, data science, and informatics to manage and analyze large datasets, facilitating information integration across levels of neural organization and scales of time and space.

Synthetic Biology and Brain Organoids

- Synthetic biology and the development of brain organoids—three-dimensional cultures that replicate aspects of brain development and function—offer new ways to study brain development, disease mechanisms, and the effects of drugs in a controlled laboratory setting. These models could revolutionize our understanding of neural circuits and the basis of neurological and psychiatric conditions.

Nanotechnology and Neuroscience

- Integrating nanotechnology into neuroscience presents opportunities to develop new imaging, sensing, and manipulating neural activity tools. Nanoscale devices could enable precise delivery of drugs to targeted brain regions or record neural activity at the level of single synapses.

Ethical Considerations

- With the advancement of brain science technologies comes a host of ethical considerations, including privacy concerns, the potential for cognitive enhancement or manipulation, and the implications of brain-computer interfacing. Addressing these ethical challenges is crucial for the responsible development and application of these technologies.

The future of cognitive neuroscience lies in integrating these emerging technologies, offering the potential to unlock the mysteries of the brain and revolutionize our approach to treating neurological disorders, enhancing cognitive function, and understanding the neural basis of human behavior.

15.2 Interdisciplinary Approaches

The complexity of the brain and the phenomena of cognition and consciousness demand a multidisciplinary approach, integrating insights from various fields to advance our understanding and develop innovative treatments. Cognitive neuroscience is inherently interdisciplinary, bridging psychology, neurology, biology, computer science, and more. Here are critical multidisciplinary approaches shaping the future of brain science and cognitive research.

Neuroengineering

- Neuroengineering combines neuroscience with engineering principles to develop technologies that interact with, understand, or mimic the nervous system. This includes the development of brain-computer interfaces (BCIs), neuroprosthetics, and devices for neural recording and stimulation. Neuroengineering aims to restore lost functions, enhance human capabilities, and deepen our understanding of how the brain processes information.

Computational Neuroscience

- Computational neuroscience uses mathematical models and theoretical analysis to understand the principles that govern brain architecture and function. Researchers can test hypotheses about brain mechanisms underlying cognition and behavior by simulating neural networks and brain systems. This approach is critical for decoding the complex dynamics of neural circuits and for developing artificial intelligence systems inspired by brain function.

Cognitive Psychology and Artificial Intelligence (AI)

- The interplay between cognitive psychology and AI is an affluent area of exploration, where insights into human cognition inform the development of intelligent systems, and computational models contribute to our understanding of cognitive processes. Machine learning, a branch of AI, has been particularly influential in modeling perception, decision-making, and language processing, offering new perspectives on learning and memory.

Genetics and Neurobiology

- Genetic and neurobiology advances have illuminated genetic factors' role in cognitive functions and neurological disorders. Techniques such as genome-wide association studies (GWAS) and CRISPR gene editing are used to identify genetic variations associated with mental traits and explore the biological pathways involved in brain development and plasticity.

Philosophy and Ethics

- Philosophy contributes to cognitive neuroscience by addressing foundational questions about the nature of consciousness, the mind-body problem, and the ethical implications of neuroscience research. As brain science technologies advance, ethical considerations regarding privacy, consent, and the impact of brain enhancement become increasingly important to address.

Social Neuroscience

- Social neuroscience examines how biological systems implement social processes and behavior, integrating methodologies from neuroscience with social psychology. This field explores the neural basis of social interactions, empathy, moral judgment, and cultural influences on cognition, emphasizing the importance of social context in brain development and function.

Neuroeconomics

- Neuroeconomics combines neuroscience, psychology, and economics to study how people make decisions, integrating the neural mechanisms involved in decision-making with economic models. This interdisciplinary approach sheds light on human behavior in financial contexts, such as risk-taking, trust, and altruism.

Interdisciplinary Collaboration

- The future of cognitive neuroscience will increasingly rely on interdisciplinary collaboration, leveraging diverse methodologies and perspectives to tackle complex questions about the brain and mind. Collaboration across disciplines fosters innovation and facilitates the translation of research findings into practical applications, from improved educational strategies to novel therapies for neurological disorders.

By embracing interdisciplinary approaches, cognitive neuroscience can advance our understanding of the brain at multiple levels, from molecular mechanisms to complex behaviors, paving the way for discoveries and technologies that enhance human health and cognitive capacities.

15.3 Ethical Considerations in Neuroscience Research

As neuroscience research advances, it raises profound ethical questions regarding the implications of these discoveries and technologies on individuals and society. Ethical considerations in neuroscience are crucial for guiding responsible research practices, protecting participants, and addressing the broader impacts of these findings. Here are critical ethical considerations in neuroscience research.

Consent and Autonomy

- **Informed Consent:** Ensuring that participants fully understand the nature, risks, and benefits of their involvement in research is fundamental. This includes studies involving vulnerable populations, such as individuals with cognitive impairments, where obtaining informed consent may be challenging.

- **Neuroethics of Emerging Technologies:** Brain-computer interfaces (BCIs) and neuroimaging raise questions about privacy and the potential misuse of neural data. Participants must be informed about how their data will be used, stored, and protected.

Cognitive Enhancement and Fairness

- The prospect of cognitive enhancement through drugs, genetic modification, or technology presents ethical dilemmas regarding access and fairness. There is a concern that such enhancements could exacerbate social inequalities or create pressure to use enhancement technologies to compete effectively in academic or professional settings.

Identity and Personality

- Interventions that potentially alter an individual's mood, personality, or cognitive functions raise questions about the impact on personal identity. Ethical considerations include respecting the individual's rights to maintain their sense of self and ensuring that interventions do not result in unwanted changes to personality or identity.

Consciousness and Animal Research

- Research on consciousness and the use of animal models in neuroscience research involves ethical considerations regarding the treatment of animals and the interpretation of findings related to consciousness in non-human subjects. Using animals in research necessitates careful, honest review to ensure humane treatment and justify the study's scientific value.

Neurological Disorders and Stigmatization

- Neuroscience research into the biological underpinnings of psychiatric and neurological disorders can contribute to reducing stigma by framing these conditions as medical issues. However, there is also a risk that natural explanations could inadvertently reinforce stigmatization by suggesting determinism or unchangeability. Ethical communication of research findings is essential to avoid misunderstanding and stigmatization.

Neuroprivacy and Cognitive Liberty

- As neuroimaging and other neurotechnologies advance, they may enable the detection of thoughts, intentions, or mental states. This raises concerns about "neuro privacy" and the right to cognitive liberty—the right of individuals to control their own cognitive and mental processes without undue influence from external technologies or interventions.

Global Ethical Standards

- The globalization of neuroscience research highlights the need for universally accepted ethical standards that respect cultural diversity while protecting participants across different contexts. Developing and adhering to international guidelines can help address ethical challenges in a globally connected research environment.

Public Engagement and Dialogue

- Engaging the public in dialogue about neuroscience research and its ethical implications is critical for building trust, understanding, and consensus on contentious issues. Public involvement can also help guide the direction of research priorities and develop policies that reflect societal values.

Addressing ethical considerations in neuroscience research requires ongoing dialogue among scientists, ethicists, policymakers, and the public. By proactively addressing these issues, the neuroscience community can ensure that research advances in a manner that respects human dignity, promotes justice, and contributes positively to society.

15.4 Exercise: 10 MCQs with Answers at the End

Test your understanding of future directions in cognitive neuroscience, including emerging technologies, interdisciplinary approaches, and ethical considerations in neuroscience research with these multiple-choice questions. Answers are provided at the end for self-assessment.

1. Optogenetics allows for the manipulation of neural activity using:

   - A) Magnetic fields

   - B) Ultrasound waves

   - C) Light

   - D) Electric currents

2. Brain-computer interfaces (BCIs) primarily aim to:

   - A) Enhance cognitive functions in healthy individuals

   - B) Create artificial intelligence systems

   - C) Establish direct communication pathways between the brain and external devices

   - D) Study the genetic basis of neurological disorders

3. High-density electroencephalography (HD-EEG) improves upon traditional EEG by offering:

- A) Lower spatial resolution

- B) Higher spatial resolution

- C) Slower data acquisition

- D) Increased invasiveness

4. The ethical principle of neuro privacy is concerned with:

- A) The equitable distribution of neurotechnologies

- B) Protecting individuals' rights to keep their neural data private

- C) Ensuring access to cognitive enhancement technologies

- D) Preventing the use of neuroimaging in research

5. Computational neuroscience utilizes _______ to understand brain function.

- A) Philosophical arguments

- B) Mathematical models

- C) Classical conditioning techniques

- D) Operant conditioning techniques

6. Neuroinformatics combines computational neuroscience with data science to:

- A) Reduce the need for empirical research

- B) Manage and analyze large datasets

- C) Eliminate ethical concerns in neuroscience

- D) Focus solely on genetic aspects of cognition

7. The concept of cognitive liberty emphasizes:

- A) The right to access cognitive enhancement technologies

- B) Freedom from government surveillance

- C) The right to control one's own cognitive and mental processes

- D) The distribution of educational resources

8. Synthetic biology and brain organoids could revolutionize our understanding of:

- A) Quantum physics

- B) Atmospheric sciences

- C) Neural circuits and neurological disorders

- D) Geological formations

9. Informed consent in neuroscience research is particularly challenging with:

- A) Healthy adult participants

- B) Animal models

- C) Vulnerable populations

- D) Computational models

10. Closed-loop stimulation systems are designed to:

- A) Monitor brain activity in real-time and deliver targeted interventions

- B) Provide continuous cognitive enhancement

- C) Record neural activity without providing feedback

- D) Stimulate brain activity randomly without monitoring

Answers:

1. C) Light

2. C) Establish direct communication pathways between the brain and external devices

3. B) Higher spatial resolution

4. B) Protecting individuals' rights to keep their neural data private

5. B) Mathematical models

6. B) Manage and analyze large datasets

7. C) The right to control one's own cognitive and mental processes

8. C) Neural circuits and neurological disorders

9. C) Vulnerable populations

10. A) Monitor brain activity in real-time and deliver targeted interventions

These questions assess your understanding of cognitive neuroscience's latest advancements and ethical challenges, highlighting the importance of interdisciplinary approaches and responsible research practices.

Conclusion

Exploring cognitive neuroscience, learning theories, and the ethical considerations of neuroscience research provides a comprehensive overview of how our understanding of the brain and cognition continues to evolve. Through the examination of principles of learning, conditioning, cognitive approaches, emerging technologies, interdisciplinary approaches, and ethical considerations, we've delved into the complexities of how we learn, think, and behave, as well as the future directions that promise to illuminate our understanding of the human mind further.

The advancements in brain science technologies, from optogenetics to brain-computer interfaces and beyond, highlight the rapid pace of innovation in the field. These technologies offer unprecedented insights into brain function and raise important ethical questions about privacy, autonomy, and the implications of cognitive enhancement.

Interdisciplinary approaches underscore the importance of integrating knowledge across various domains—combining insights from psychology, neurology, computer science, engineering, and ethics—to tackle the brain's complexities. This collaborative effort is crucial for advancing our understanding of cognitive processes and developing effective treatments for neurological disorders.

Ethical considerations remind us of the responsibility that comes with advancing knowledge. As we continue to explore the frontiers of brain science, maintaining a focus on ethical research practices, informed consent, cognitive liberty, and equitable access to technologies will ensure that the benefits of discoveries are shared broadly and contribute positively to society.

In conclusion, the journey through cognitive neuroscience and related disciplines reveals a vibrant, challenging field full of potential. As we look to the future, continued curiosity, ethical vigilance, and interdisciplinary collaboration will be vital to unlocking the mysteries of the brain and enhancing human cognitive capacities in responsible and meaningful ways.

*The best way to thank an author is
to
write a review.*